TAI CHI SECRETS OF THE
ANCIENT MASTERS

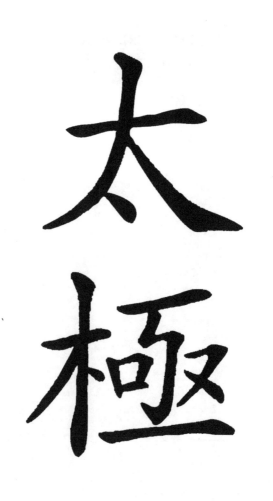

TAI CHI SECRETS
of the
ANCIENT MASTERS

*Selected Readings
with Commentary*

太極拳先哲秘要

Translation & Commentary
by Dr. Yang, Jwing-Ming

YMAA Publication Center
Wolfeboro, NH USA

Publisher's Cataloging-in-Publication
(Provided by Quality Books, Inc.)

Tai chi secrets of the ancient masters : selected readings
    with commentary / translation & commentary by
    Dr. Yang, Jwing-Ming. – 1st ed.
       p. cm. – (Tai chi treasures ; 2)
       LCCN: 98-61694
       ISBN: 1-886969-71-X

    1. Chinese poetry. 2. T'ai ch'i ch'uan–Poetry.
  I. Yang, Jwing-Ming, 1946-

PL2518.8.M37Y36 1999   895.1'1
                          QBI98-1723

YMAA Publication Center
PO Box 480
Wolfeboro, NH 03894
www.ymaa.com • info@ymaa.com

Foreword

The wisdom of Taijiquan is precious, and that is why it was kept in secrecy for so many centuries. In this way, the more exact memory of how to so fully enrich and protect life has been practiced and preserved. Now, the secrets are being opened for us. A comparison of the poetry of Taijiquan, to the poems of European and even other Asiatic civilizations, reveals the unique qualities that make the Taiji poems both instructive and heraldic of mystery.

Poetry is often given to the poet by the deliberate forces of life, the forces of a rare and difficult talent, in a lifetime where wisdom is essential to this talent. Poetry is the gift of painting and singing the emotions, what these Taijiquan secret poems refer to as heart and mind. European poetry and culture do not have such a subject as Taiji, a military art that offers spiritual enlightenment and transcendence—the sublime. However, for all their differences, traditions in European poetry and Chinese poetry—secret or esoteric in whatever degree—both broadly celebrate the effort to live, to love.

Anna Akhmatova, the great Russian poet, wrote these lines in "Requiem":

The mountains bend before this grief
The great river does not flow
But the prison locks are strong.

This could have been a comment on Taiji Push Hands, but that was not Akhmatova's intention. It is instead meant for the suffering and the dead in the Stalinist Soviet Union. In the same way, Homer's Iliad and Odyssey have the emotive and evocative power in imagery drawn from nature, images which may remind one of the uses of nature in Taijiquan poems. Still, it is more the lyric poem in European writing that approaches the feeling of Taijiquan poetry, lyric poems such as those of Akhmatova or John Dunne, to name just two. As feelings are the palette of both the Western lyric and Taijiquan, it is here where the two poetic traditions have a common meeting place, a communion.

In the Taijiquan secret poems, we see all life being celebrated in the practice of the art, perhaps the greater part of life in the solo form. The names of the postures themselves have the evocative power of poetry. Witness Fair Lady Works at the Shuttles, or Grasp Sparrow's Tail. In these poems, a single word carries the wisdom and practice of many generations, all of them convinced of the body's innate wisdom. The Taijiquan secret poetry tells us to love and cherish life, both as it is revealed to us through our practice, and as it is further hidden as our understanding deepens.

The poet Stephen Shu-ning Liu writes in his poem "My Father's Martial Art" these words:

> ...don't retreat into night, my father
> Come down from the cliffs...

Dr. Yang Jwing-Ming has brought the secrets from the cliffs.

Afaa Michael Weaver
November, 1998

Introduction

In the last seven centuries, many songs and poems have been composed about Taijiquan. These have played a major role in preserving the knowledge and wisdom of the masters, although in many cases the identity of the authors and the dates of origin have been lost. Since many Chinese people of previous centuries were illiterate, many of the key points of the art were put into poems and songs, which are easier to remember than prose, and passed down orally from teacher to student. Treatises, which usually are more profound than the poems and songs, were also passed down. These documents were regarded as secret, and it was only in the twentieth century that they were revealed to the general public.

Almost all of the documents currently available can be categorized into four groups. The first group is the most general; it includes the most ancient documents, written either by known or unknown authors, and also those authors who do not belong to a specific style. The second of these four groups is comprised of those poems, songs, or treatises passed down by ancestors of Yang, Chen, and Wu families. This small book will introduce the first group with twenty-one poems, songs, and treatises. Many of these are considered the most popular of their kind, and are the most accurate in presenting the art of Taijiquan. In the near future, the other groups of documents will be translated and presented in similar fashion.

It should come as no surprise to the reader that it is very difficult to translate ancient Chinese writings into modern English. Because of the cultural differences, many expressions simply do not make any sense, if translated literally. Often, knowledge of the historical context is necessary. Furthermore, since every sound has several possible meanings, anybody who has ever tried to reduce these poems to writing has had to choose from among these different meanings. Over the course of several generations, this has led to variation among the poems. The same problem occurs when the poems are read. Many Chinese characters have several possible meanings, so reading involves interpretation of the text, even for the Chinese. Also, the meaning of many words has changed over the course of time. When you add to this the grammatical differences (generally, no tenses, no articles, no distinction between singular and plural, and no differentiation between parts of speech) it becomes almost impossible to provide a literal translation from Chinese to English.

With these difficulties in mind, I have attempted to convey as much of the original meaning of the Chinese as possible, based on my own thirty-seven years of Taiji experience and understanding. Although it is impossible to totally translate the original meaning, I feel that I have managed to express the majority of the important points. The translation has been made as close to the original Chinese as possible, including such things as double negatives and, sometimes, idiosyncratic sentence structure. Words that are understood but not actually written in the Chinese text have been included in parentheses. Also, some Chinese words are followed by the English in parentheses, e.g. Shen (Spirit) and some English words are followed by original Chinese, e.g. Essence (Jing). To further assist the reader, I have included commentary with each poem, song, and treatise. For your further reference, the original Chinese of each document is included in Appendix A. In addition, a glossary of Chinese terms is included in Appendix B for your convenience.

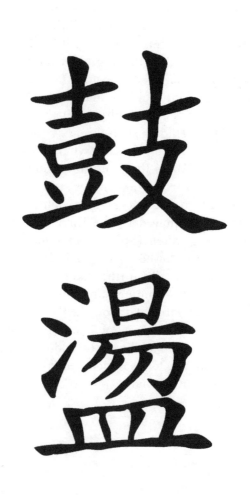

鼓

盪

1. Taijiquan Treatise[1,5]
by Zhang, San-Feng

Once in motion,
Entire body must be light (Qing) and agile
* (Ling),*
(It) especially should (be) threaded together.

Qing Ling, the Chinese words that are translated "light and agile," are used to describe the movement of monkeys: responsive, controlled, and able to move quickly. This line implies that the body's movement must be soft, relaxed, smooth, natural, and comfortable. When this happens, there is no body tightness, no stagnation of Qi, and no mental confusion. Softness will enter into your every motion, and you will move naturally, quickly and efficiently.

The body should be a coherent whole, with all of its parts connected and unified by the energy (Qi) moving within them, like ancient Chinese coins connected by a string. Taiji Jin (martial power) is classified as a soft Jin. In order to manifest soft Jin, the body must act like a soft whip to express the power forward. All of the joints must be soft and relaxed. The muscles on the limbs and in the

1

torso must also remain relaxed. You must practice the movements until they feel completely natural and effortless. If the muscles and the joints are tensed, then the Jin manifested will be hard, and will not penetrate. Such hard power is not a characteristic of Taijiquan.

Qi should be full and stimulated (Gu Dang), Shen (Spirit) should be retained internally.

In Chinese, Gu Dang means a drum that is full and resounding (due to vibration). The Qi that is generated and stored in the Lower Dan Tian should be full, like an air filled drum which can produce powerful vibrations. When your Qi is full and stored in the Lower Dan Tian, your life energy will be strong. Consequently, the Qi led by the mind through the body will be abundant, and your Jin will be powerful. In order to store the Qi abundantly, you must learn Embryo Breathing (Tai Xi), and in order to lead the Qi to the entire body, you must learn Small Circulation and Grand Circulation meditation. Such purely internal work, performed independently of your form practice, will enable you to apply the principles into your Taiji.

Doing Taiji practice, although the Qi is full and stimulated, your mind is centered and controlled, so that the Qi doesn't scatter.

Retaining the Spirit of Vitality internally means to be calm, patient, and restrained in your actions. This helps to avoid giving away your intentions to your partner, and conserves your Qi. When the spirit is retained internally, the mind will be concentrated and controlled.

No part should be defective,
No part should be deficient or excessive,
And no part should be disconnected.

This sentence stresses the importance of accuracy in the movements (or postures). Taijiquan is an internal martial art. In order to protect yourself effectively and manifest your Jin efficiently, you must stand and move with balance, efficiency, and precision. Your mind must sink the body down, into the floor. This sinking will help you to manifest your intention clearly and without tensing your body. No posture or part of the body should stretch out too far or be pulled in too much. Every motion should be smooth, always just right; your strength applied just enough to do the job, and a little bit held in reserve. In addition, each posture should be rounded and should involve the whole body in a smooth, continuous, flowing motion.

The root is at the feet,
(Jin or movement is) generated from the legs,
Mastered (i.e., controlled) by the waist

3

And manifested (i.e., expressed) from the fingers.
From the feet to the legs to the waist must be
*   integrated, and one unified Qi.*
When moving forward or backward,
(You can) then catch the opportunity and gain
*   the superior position.*

When performing Jin in your Taiji practice, your entire body acts like a soft whip. By sinking down and settling your mind, you become rooted. Once you have a firm root, the legs are able to generate the motion or Jin (martial power). This power can then be directed by the waist, and manifested from the hands to the target as desired. The waist is thus like the steering wheel of a car, guiding the direction of your power like the wheels of a car. If you are firmly connected to the ground, and connected from the feet to the waist, you can move as a coherent unit. Then, your Jin will be strong, and you will be agile and responsive enough to gain an advantageous position.

The Qi of the entire body must be unified in the technique. It is important to balance the force and Qi of the substantial (active) hand with the root in the feet, and to balance the insubstantial force suspending the head with the Qi sunk to the Dan Tian. The trick to unifying the Qi and the techniques is correct Taijiquan breathing.

If you fail to catch the opportunity
and gain the superior position,
(your) body will be disordered.
To solve this problem,
(you) must look to the waist and legs.

If you do not catch the right timing and
opportunity for your attack or defense, your
mind can be scattered and your body unbal-
anced and disorganized. When this happens,
your root will be shallow and infirm. When
your root is not firm, you lose the foundation
through which the legs generate power.
Consequently, your waist loses control, and
its actions become meaningless. Your energy
will become disconnected, and you will begin
to float upward, out of your root. To remedy
this, you must properly align your waist and
legs, enabling you to rebuild your root and
stabilize yourself. Also, bring your mind back
to your breathing, making it once again deep,
slow, soft and uniform. Make this a continuous process. Constantly bring your senses to
the proper breathing and body alignment.

This is especially rewarding during pushing hands practice. If your partner places you
in an awkward position, or is dynamically
moving you into an unfavorable situation,
your body will often tense, which allows your
partner to find your center and "root-push"
you off balance. Whenever you discover yourself entering such a position or situation, if

you immediately lower your body to re-root through your foundation, while using your breathing and your waist to neutralize the incoming manifestation of energy, you are frequently able to change your positioning, and neutralize your partner's control.

> Up and down, forward and backward, left and
>   right,
> It's all the same.
> All of this is done with the Yi (mind),
> Not externally.

The Chinese believe that there are two minds. One mind is called Xin (i.e., heart or emotional mind) and the other is called Yi (wisdom mind). The emotional mind (i.e., Yang mind) acts like a monkey, jumping around, unsteady, excited easily, emotional and fun loving, while the wisdom mind (Yin mind) behaves like a horse, very powerful, yet controlled. When you encounter hostility, your wisdom mind with wise judgment should control instead of the emotional mind. Look beneath the surface to discover true motivations.

For any direction, with any motion, it always comes down to adjusting the waist and legs. You do not rely on quick, forceful motions of the body or arms. Instead, the mind perceives the situation and the most effective solution, and it directs the body. All of this depends on the sensitivity of your listening Jin, where you attempt to use your mind to sense the energy of the situation, and to move in harmony with that perceived energy. This mind and body coordination can only be achieved through consistent, dedicated practice of the art with an appreciation of the natural world.

If there is a top, there is a bottom;
If there is a front, there is a back;
If there is a left, there is a right.

The first meaning of this sentence is to keep your body centered. When up and down, left and right, front and back are balanced, you will be centered. When you are centered, you can build up a firm root.

When you are centered, your mind will be on the Lower Dan Tian, and the Qi can be gathered there abundantly. When you are centered, you are able to use your waist to direct the action and power easily and smoothly.

The second meaning of this sentence is to have living strategic movements. Taijiquan emphasizes completeness; when attacking high, you must defend low; when moving in one direction, you must balance mind and Qi in the opposite direction; when attacking or defending on one side, you must be aware of the other side.

The third meaning of this sentence is to manifest the Jin with balanced power. Balancing your energy is a crucial key to effective offensive and defensive Jin manifestation. If you can grasp the trick of this balance, you will understand the secret of Jin manifestation.

If Yi (wisdom mind) wants to go upward,
This implies considering downward.
(This means) if (you) want to lift and defeat an
   opponent,
You must first consider his root.
When the opponent's root is broken,
He will inevitably be defeated quickly and cer-
   tainly.

Your partner's root is his foundation. When his root is broken, he will lose his foundation and his Jin will not be generated from the legs and controlled by the waist. This will greatly limit his fighting ability. If you wish to knock him down or push him away, you must first break his root so that he is unstable and can be easily defeated. In addition, when your partner loses his root, his mind temporarily will be scattered and confused, and this will provide you with a good opportunity to attack.

Substantial and insubstantial must be clearly
   distinguished.
Every part (of the body)
Has a substantial and an insubstantial aspect.

*The entire body and all the joints should be
threaded together without the slightest break.*

It is very important to distinguish between
substantial and insubstantial in your body and
in your partner's. The hand acting upon your
partner is substantial, while the other hand is
insubstantial. The leg with more weight on it
is usually substantial, but an insubstantial leg
(such as the front leg in the false stance)
becomes substantial upon kicking. When
pushing, the front of the hand is substantial,
while the back of the hand is insubstantial.
You must also clearly distinguish and respond
to your partner's substantial and insubstantial.
When your partner attacks your right side, that
side should become insubstantial, and your
left side should become substantial to attack
him. In order to do all this effectively, your
entire body—from the feet, legs and waist to
the fingers—must work like a unit, and move
as if threaded together, like a soft whip.

Following are additional sentences from
Zhang, San-Feng.[1] However, there are some
documents which attribute them to Wang,
Zon-Yue.[4,5]

What is Long Fist?
(It is) like a long river and a large ocean,
Rolling ceaselessly.

There are two styles of martial arts in China called "Long Fist" (Chang Quan). One is Taijiquan, in which case "Chang Quan" is translated "Long Sequence." This is because the Taiji sequence is long, and the movements are performed smoothly and continuously like a flowing river. The other "Chang Quan" is translated as "Long Fist," and refers to a northern external style that emphasizes long range fighting strategies.

What are the thirteen patterns (Shi)?
Peng (Wardoff), Lu (Rollback), Ji (Press), An (Push),
Cai (Pluck), Lie (Split), Zhou (Elbow), Kao (Bump),
These are the eight trigrams.
Jin Bu (Forward), Tui Bu (Backward), Zuo Gu (Beware of the Left), You Pan (Look to the Right), Zhong Ding (Central Equilibrium, or Firmness),
These are the five elements.
Wardoff, Rollback, Press, and Push are Qian (Heaven), Kun (Earth), Kan (Water), Li (Fire), the four main sides.
Pluck, Split, Elbow, Bump are Xun (Wind), Zhen (Thunder), Dui (Lake), and Gen (Mountain), the four diagonal corners.
Forward, Backward, Beware of the Left, Look to the right, and Central Equilibrium (or Firmness) are Jin (Metal), Mu (Wood), Shui (Water), Huo (Fire), and Tu (Earth).
All together they are the thirteen patterns (Shi).

In this sentence, the first thing that must be clear in your mind is that the Chinese word "Shi," though commonly translated as "postures," has the meanings of "appearance," "way," "situation," "patterns" or some object or subject. Therefore, the more accurate translation of "Shi" here should be patterns. It is from these patterns that many postures are derived.

This paragraph lists Taiji's basic moving patterns and their correlates. Taijiquan is also called "thirteen patterns." This is because Taijiquan is constructed from eight fundamental basic strategic moving patterns and five maneuvering stepping techniques. The eight patterns are also called "Eight Doors" (Ba Men) and the five steppings are called, not surprisingly, "Five Steppings" (Wu Bu). All of these are called the "Thirteen Patterns" of Taijiquan.

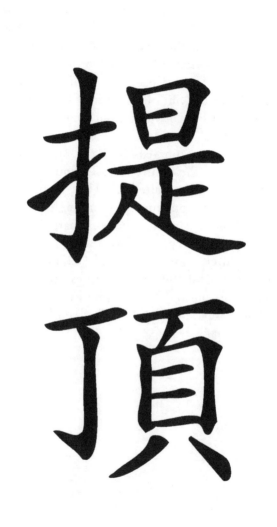

2. Taijiquan Classic[1-5]
by Wang, Zong-Yue

What is Taiji?
It is generated from Wuji,
And is a pivotal function of movement and still-
ness.
It is the mother of Yin and Yang.
When it moves, it divides. At rest it reunites.

Taiji can be translated as "Grand Ultimate," or "Grand Extremity," and Wuji is translated as "Without Ultimate," "Without Limit," or "No Extremity." Wuji can also mean "No Opposition." This means Wuji is uniform and undifferentiated, a point in space at the center of your physical, mental and energetic bodies. For example, at the beginning of the universe, for a very, very short period of time, there was no differentiation, and this state is called Wuji. Within the first microseconds, the universe began its separation into complimentary opposites, called Yin and Yang. From the interaction of Yin and Yang, all things are generated and grow.

This Wuji state still exists inside each of us. It is the state from which all creative impulses grow. Taiji is generated out of Wuji. Taiji is the cause of Yin and Yang division, and itself is neither Wuji nor Yin and Yang, but the cause of the Yin and Yang's separation. In this sense it is a part of the divine aspect of the Dao.

All objects, ideas, spirits, etc. can be identified as either Yin or Yang. Taijiquan was created according to this theory. In the beginning posture of the Taiji sequence, the mind is calm and empty, and the weight is evenly distributed on both feet. This state is Wuji. As soon as your mind leads the body into Grasp Sparrow's Tail, the hands and feet differentiate into substantial and insubstantial. The interaction of substantial (Yang) and insubstantial (Yin) generates all of Taijiquan's fighting strategy and technique. From this, you can see the that the Taiji (i.e., the Dao) in Taijiquan is actually the mind. It is the mind that makes the body move, and Wuji divide.

No excess, no deficiency.
Following (the opponent), bend, then extend.

No part of your posture should be exaggerated or constricted, nothing should be too concave or too convex. When you stick to and follow your partner, do only what is appropriate — no more, no less. In pushing hands, when your partner pushes your arm, yield. Adhere lightly to his arm, following his motion with no separation or resistance.

14

When he attacks, give way elastically, and when he withdraws, extend to follow him.

When the opponent is hard, I am soft;
This is called yielding.
When I follow the opponent,
This is called adhering.

When your partner attacks you, do not resist him, but instead give way and lead his force into emptiness, so that his attack misses you. The Chinese term translated as "yielding" literally means "walk away." Adhering to your partner means to maintain contact with him and follow his motions, so that when the right time comes, you can make the appropriate move.

When the opponent moves fast, I move fast;
When the opponent moves slowly, then I follow
   slowly.
Although the variations are infinite,
   the principle remains the same.

The principle here, as in the previous two sections, is to adhere to your partner and follow his motions. You can then respond appropriately no matter what he does. Although there are many techniques, they are all variations on the one basic principle of adhering and following.

*After you have mastered (the techniques of
  adhering and following),
Then you can gradually grasp what
  "Understanding Jin (Dong Jin)" means.
From "Understanding Jin," you gradually
  approach enlightenment (intuitive understanding) of your opponent's intention.
However, without a great deal of study over a
  long time, you cannot grasp this intuitive
  understanding of your opponent.*

When you have grasped the key to adhering and following, you should master them
and make them skillful enough to apply into
the various techniques. Then you can begin
to understand your partner's Jin, and can
interpret his intentions. The more you practice, the more sensitive you will become.

*An insubstantial energy leads the head upward.
The Qi is sunk to the Dan Tian.*

An insubstantial energy lifts the head
upward so that it feels like the head and body
are suspended by a string attached to the top
of the head. This energy is balanced by the Qi
sunk to the Dan Tian and the bottom of the
feet. When the head is upright, the Spirit of
Vitality will be raised, alertness will increase,
and the body will be straight and erect from
the tailbone to the top of the head. When the
Qi is sunk to the Dan Tian, the mind is calm,
and the root is strengthened.

No tilting, no leaning.
Suddenly disappear, suddenly appear.

The head and body are balanced upright. Do not tilt your body in any direction. If you maintain a relaxed, centered, and balanced posture, and adhere and follow, you can respond easily and lightly to your partner. You then can "disappear" in front of your partner's attack, and "appear" with your own attack where he doesn't expect you.

When there is pressure on the left, the left
*   becomes insubstantial;*
When there is pressure on the right, the right
*   becomes insubstantial.*
Looking upward it seems to get higher and
*   higher;*
Looking downward it seems to get deeper and
*   deeper.*
When (the opponent) advances, it seems longer
*   and longer;*
When (the opponent) retreats, it becomes more
*   and more urgent.*
A feather cannot be added and a fly cannot
*   land.*
The opponent does not know me, but I know the
*   opponent.*
A hero has no equal because of all of this.

Wherever your partner attacks, that part of you withdraws. When he tries to reach you, you fade away, just out of range of his power. When he tries to withdraw, you adhere to him like glue. He feels that you are right there pushing him, and he can't get away. No matter what he does, you adhere and follow. After much practice, you can be so sensitive and accurate in your response that not even a feather can touch you without setting you in motion. Your partner can never catch hold of you to figure you out, but you always know him. If you reach this level, no one can match you. In order to reach this level, you must train listening Jin (i.e., skin feeling and sensitivity). Skin feeling is a tool for communication between your body and your partner's. If you can build up high enough sensitivity, you will have the capability to control your partner as you wish.

> *Although in techniques, there are many side*
>   *doors (i.e., other martial art styles),*
> *And the postures are distinguishable from one*
>   *another,*
> *After all, it is nothing more than the strong*
>   *beating the weak,*
> *The slow yielding to the fast.*
> *The one with power beats the one without*
>   *power,*
> *The slow hands yield to the fast hands.*
> *All this is natural born ability.*
> *It is not related to the power that has to be*
>   *learned.*

Taijiquan is different from most other Gongfu styles in which one uses his natural born abilities of strength and speed to defend one's self. Taijiquan is an internal martial art which uses the mind to lead the Qi for power manifestation. Its power can be very soft, yet can be deadly. It's moving can be slow, yet your partner is under control. All of this relies on the training of internal sensitivity and power, and their coordination with the external postures. Reaching this stage not only takes time, patience, and perseverance to learn the skills and techniques, but also requires talent and a comprehending mind to understand the theory, strategy, and approach.

> Investigate (consider) the saying: "Four ounces repel one thousand pounds."
> It is apparent that this cannot be accomplished by strength.
> Look, if an eighty or ninety-year old man can still defend himself against multiple opponents,
> It cannot be a matter of speed.

Taijiquan teaches you to rely on technique and an understanding of your partner, rather than mere strength or speed. After doing the sequence correctly for many years, your body will be healthy and you will have built up internal energy, which is quite different from external strength. If you understand the principles of neutralizing, adhering and sticking, and if you have practiced Taiji pushing hands and applications for many years, you can fight effectively even when you are old.

*Stand like a balanced scale, (move) lively like a
   cartwheel.*

The body stands upright, centered and in
equilibrium, just like a scale balancing two
weights. Neutralize incoming forces by moving your whole body as a unit, with the cen-
terline of your body acting as the axle.

*(When the opponent presses) sideward (or)
   downward, then follow.*
*(When there is) double heaviness (mutual resis-
   tance), then (there is) stagnation.*
*Often, after several years of dedicated training,
   one still cannot apply this neutralization and
   is controlled by the opponent.*
*(The reason for this is that the) fault of double
   heaviness is not understood.*

Whether your partner attacks high or low,
left or right, you do not resist him. Instead,
you yield and follow, adhering to him
patiently until you have a good opportunity
to attack. If you struggle against him, the
liveliness of the interaction stagnates, and
victory will go to the one with the most external strength. In Taiji, the attacking hand is
considered "heavy" because it is putting
weight or pressure on your partner. The
Chinese character Zhong can be translated
as "weight" and Shuang as "pair" or "double."
Therefore, some authors translate Shuang
Zhong as "double weighting." However, the

same character Zhong can also be pronounced Chong, translated as "repeated overlapping." Therefore, Shuang Chong can be translated as "double overlapping." This means "mutual covering and resistance" and has the sense of two forces struggling against each other, each striving for the upper hand. If you study for many years, but never grasp the importance of avoiding this "mutual resistance," then you will never get the knack of neutralizing your partner's energy.

> To avoid this fault (you) must know Yin and
> Yang.
> To adhere means to yield. To yield means to
> adhere.
> Yin not separate from Yang. Yang not separate
> from Yin.
> Yin and Yang mutually cooperate, (understanding this) is "Understanding Jin" (Dong Jin).

You must thoroughly internalize the principle of always yielding to your partner's attack while remaining lightly attached to him. Your Yin defense is dependent upon and interrelated to his Yang attack. When you have neutralized his attack, your Yin becomes Yang as you attack. If you always stay in contact with your partner and carefully pay attention (listen) to his motion and Jin (energy), you will gradually develop the ability to understand his intention. Once you learn how extreme Yin becomes Yang and extreme

Yang becomes Yin, you will learn the knack of timing your attacks and defense, and will gain the ability to "borrow" your partner's force. When you know these things, you know Understanding Jin.

> *After Understanding Jin, the more practice, the more refinement.*
> *Silently learn, then ponder; gradually you will approach your heart's desire.*

Once you master Understanding Jin, the more you practice, the more you will progress. Your own study and experience, during which you ponder silently in your own mind, is your main source of improvement. If you follow this method you can eventually reach the highest levels of achievement, where whatever you wish is done naturally.

> *Fundamentally, give yourself up and follow the opponent.*
> *Many misunderstand and give up the near for the far.*
> *This means a slight error can cause a thousand-mile divergence.*
> *The learner, therefore, must discriminate precisely.*

The most important principle is to give yourself up, and follow the other person. This does not mean becoming totally passive and just meekly following him. Stick and follow patiently and conscientiously, and when an opportunity presents itself, attack. If instead you try this and that to attack your partner, or actively try to get him in a bad position, this is called "giving up the near for the far."

It is important for the student to be very discriminating in determining what is right and wrong, because a small error of principle in the beginning of training will have greater and greater consequences as time goes on.

> *Every sentence in this thesis is important.*
> *Not a single word has been added carelessly, or*
>   *for decoration.*
> *(Those) without a high degree of wisdom won't*
>   *be able to understand.*
> *The past teachers were not willing to teach*
>   *indiscriminately,*
> *Not just because of (the difficulty of) choosing*
>   *people,*
> *But also because they were afraid of wasting*
>   *their time and energy.*

The Taiji classics describe a very high level of awareness and understanding. Each description is an attempt to bring the reader closer to the principles of Taiji and to the experiences of the author. No part can be separated from the others, and nothing can be omitted. The author arrived at his understanding through long and arduous effort, and anyone wishing to learn this art must be willing and able to match this effort.

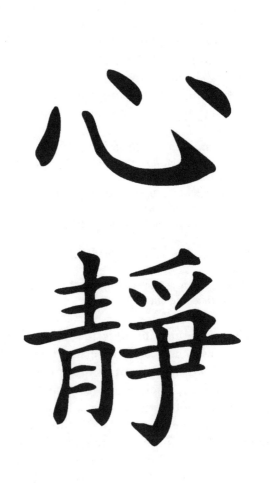

3. Four Important Sentences[6]
by Yang, Yu-Ting

*The joints must be loose, the skin and hair must
be attacked (i.e., reached by Qi),
Section and section threaded together, insubstantial and dexterity is within.*

In order to be soft, you must first relax. In
order to be relaxed, your joints must first
loosen. When the joints are loose, you can
move your body as one unit and manifest your
Jin like a soft whip.

To manifest Jin effectively, you must first
have abundant Qi circulating in your body.
Moreover, you must know to lead the Qi to
the skin surface, to enhance Guardian Qi
through skin breathing (Ti Xi). When your
guardian Qi is strong, you can build up the
sensitivity of the skin. When this happens,
your listening Jin will reach a high level.
Listening Jin must be developed first, followed by following and adhering Jin.

In addition, in order to manifest Taiji Jin
softly, you must be attentive to the joints in
your body. Any joint in your body is constructed from two or more bones, connected by
ligaments. If the joint is twisted, overextended,

or turned in a manner contrary to its design, the ligaments will be damaged, and the joint will become stiff and inflamed. Jin training and pushing hands are the most common types of Taijiquan practice which can produce injuries in a practitioner. The ligaments and tendons must be conditioned to avoid injury when soft Jin is emitted. Furthermore, in order to generate Jin from the root, governed by the waist, and manifested at the hands, you must treat the entire body as a single unit (i.e., a soft whip). All of the joints must be threaded together without any breaks. Only then can your Jin be manifested efficiently and skillfully.

There are several training techniques for building up the Qi to an abundant level, and for learning how to lead this stored Qi to different parts of your body. Sitting meditation can help you to build the Qi in your Dan Tian, and allows you to use only your mind and breathing to move the Qi through the Governing and Conception Vessels. Sitting meditation and moving Qigong can lead you to discover how to move the Qi in order to support your physical movements. Coiling Qigong will assist you in building up the sensitivity of your skin, and will improve the health and flexibility of your joints. Proper Taijiquan and push hands training should incorporate Taiji form training, Qigong and still meditation. Care should also be taken to incorporate some form of endurance training as well.

If you can fulfill the above conditions, your movements will be agile and your spirit of vitality will be high. You will begin to feel that your Taiji practice goes beyond simple form training, and you will be able to perceive things as energetic combinations, rather than as static physical objects. Your training partners will appear to your senses as dynamic patterns of energy, rather than as clumsy physical bodies. When this happens, you can skillfully switch strategy and tactics in any situation. You will know your partner and your partner will not know you. This is what is meant by your dexterity coming from within.

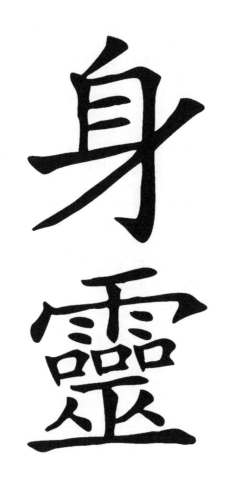

4. Thirteen Important Keys of Regulating the Body[2]
by Gu, Liu-Xing

1. Xin (i.e., emotional mind) calms, use Yi. The body upright and loose.

Xin is the emotional mind, which acts like a monkey, while Yi is the wisdom mind, which can be powerful yet controlled, like a horse. In combat, you cannot be overwhelmed by your emotional mind. If you fight only with your emotional mind, you will lose control of yourself both spiritually and physically. When the emotional mind is calm, your mind is clear and the judgment will be accurate.

In order to have clear judgment in a fight, you must be relaxed and not tensed. The key to this is to keep your body centered, and all of the joints loose. When this happens, your mind and physical body will be centered, and your thinking will not be confused and scattered.

2. From loose to soft. Within the softness, resides the hardness.

In order to manifest Taiji Jin as softly as a whip, you must first learn how to be loose. All the joints are threaded together, and are loosely connected. Only if you can manifest the Jin softly will your power be penetrating and focused for cavity attacks. Cavity strikes can shock the internal organs and cause significant damage. Therefore, though the Jin is soft, its damage is hard.

3. *Curving shape and spiral (i.e., coil), (the mind and the body) are centered and the (Qi) body is round.*

In Taijiquan, in order to change the strategy from insubstantial to substantial and vice versa, you must be skillful in the technique of coiling. Coiling is a spiral movement which allows you to change the techniques from Yin to Yang and from Yang to Yin. Moreover, once you grasp the trick of coiling, your hands will always be on the top of your partner's limbs to govern the entire condition. When this happens, you put your partner into a defensive situation.

In order to have skillful spiraling movements, the mind and body must be centered. In addition, you should always keep the body in a rounded state (i.e., Peng Jin). When your body is in a good Peng Jin state, your partner will not be able to connect with your center easily. The coiling techniques must be done with the entire body, instead of just using your arms. To reach this goal, your body must move with round and circling patterns. Only in the round movements can coiling be efficient.

> 4. *The movements are originated from waist and spine, the Jin reaches the four extremities.*

Although the Jins are generated from the legs, this is only a source of power. In addition, all of the correspondence to your partner's actions must be performed by the waist and spine. The waist is the steering wheel of the Jin, which directs the emitted Jin and also neutralizes incoming Jin. The spine is a large bow, constructed from two bows of reversing curvature. If you can respond to an incoming attack skillfully with your waist and torso, you will have grasped the trick of directing the Jins.

Even if you can direct the Jin, if it cannot reach to your fingers, your effort is still in vain. When this happens, all of the power remains in your body, and eventually, this will harm you. Correct Jin emission directs the Jin to your partner's body. Your mental target should be about six inches beyond your hands. Only then will your Jin be useful and effective.

This sentence emphasizes the importance of the waist and torso.

> 5. *Three points and six unified (harmonized), the up and bottom is one line.*

The three points are the tip of the nose, the fingers, and the toes. In most of the Taijiquan postures, the finger tips and the tip of the nose should line up horizontally. Also, the finger tips of the front hand and the tips of the front toes should line up vertically. When these three tips are lined up correctly, it establishes a firm posture for both defense and offense. Your breathing (i.e., nose) is coordinated with the stepping (i.e., feet) and hand techniques (i.e., fingers). Therefore, you harmonize the three points internally as well.

Six unifications means the unification of the two hands and the two feet, the two elbows and two knees, and the two shoulders and the two hips. When these are unified, the movements from the top to the bottom will be coordinated, and you will be centered.

When all of this happens, the top of your head (Baihui) and your perineum (Huiyin or Haidi) will be vertically aligned. You will be centered and balanced. Once you attain this center and balance, you can build a firm root and raise the spirit of vitality.

> 6. *Insubstantial (energy) leads the head upward, the Qi is sunk to the (Lower) Dan Tian.*

To raise the Spirit of Vitality (i.e., Yang manifestation), the body should be upright and the head should be led upward, as if there were an invisible energy lifting it upward. The Yin side of this energy is to sink the Qi to the Lower Dan Tian. If you can comprehend this Yin and Yang balance both externally and internally, you will grasp one of the most subtle secrets of Taijiquan.

   7. *Swallow the chest and stretch the back. Drop*
      the Kua (i.e., inner thighs) and collapse the
      waist.

Swallow the chest and stretch the back is an action of Peng (i.e., Wardoff). From this action, you can yield to incoming force while you store Jin in your posture (i.e., chest and spine). In addition, you should firm the inner thighs (Kua), which builds up the connection from the body to the root in the legs. Collapse the waist means to loosen the waist. Since the waist directs the power, it must be soft and loose.

   8. *Drop the elbow and sink the shoulder. Settle*
      the wrist and soothe the fingers.

When you drop the elbow and sink the shoulder, the Jin manifested from your upper limbs will be rooted, allowing you to connect your arms to your body, and root it to the ground. If your elbows are lifted and your shoulders are raised, the Jin manifested will be from your arms, and not from your body.

When you manifest your Jin from your palms, at the beginning your wrists and your fingers are extremely relaxed and comfortable. This allows the Qi to reach your palms easily. However, just before you reach your partner's body, settle your wrist to firm your palm, so that the power can be strongly emitted, without injury to yourself. "Settle the Wrist" is the key word of An (i.e., press or push downward, upward, forward).

> 9. Bend the knee and open (the) groin, the hip bone has strength.

When the knees are bent, your knees will not be locked, remaining loose and easily moved. If your knees are locked, your stepping will be stagnant and slow. The groin area should be open so the Huiyin cavity (i.e., perineum) will be relaxed and loose. This will allow the Qi to circulate smoothly in the Small and Grand circulation. Moreover, when the groin is open, the waist and lower back will be relaxed. When this happens, your root will be firmed and the waist can be used to direct the Jin smoothly and easily. However, even with the groin area loose and relaxed, the hips must be strong, firmly connecting the torso to the legs. Otherwise, your root will be shallow. A firm root originates from strong hips.

10. The eyes are turned following the hands,
exchanging the steps following the body.

When you are in combat, before any physical contact, the eyes connect with your partner. When the eyes can collect every subtle action of your partner's movement, and this information can be relayed to the brain instantly, without any type of internal dialogue whatsoever, then you will enter a completely alert state. Your spirit will be raised to a high level, to the point where your partner can actually feel it overcoming him. However, once contact is established, you must use listening (i.e., feeling), understanding, and adhering Jin. At this point, your skin's sensitivity becomes extremely important. Once the physical contact is broken, the eyes are again of primary importance. The eyes follow the hands for intercepting and blocking.

In combat, the stepping must follow your body's movement, and your body's movement follows the strategic situation. All action must correspond with your partner's intention. Therefore, you must practice with a partner until all of the body movements and stepping techniques naturally and automatically follow the strategic situation.

11. Speed is uniform, light and sunken (i.e.,
heavy) both required.

When you perform the Taiji sequence, the speed should be uniform, which allows you to harmoniously coordinate your breathing and your mind with the movements. It is very important that you learn to use your mind to lead the Qi downward to establish a firm root (i.e., heavy). However, it is equally important that, once you decide to move your feet, you are agile and light.

Once you have achieved a profound level of Taijiquan practice, you start to build up a sense of enemy. When this happens, the speed of your actions depends upon your enemy. When he is fast, you are fast, and when he is slow, you follow slow. When he is heavy (i.e., heavy force), you can be light, and when he is light, you can become heavy.

12. Initiate internally and emit externally, the breathing is harmonious.

Whenever you decide to take action, first the Yi (i.e., wisdom mind) is generated. This mind leads the Qi (i.e., bioelectricity) to the physical body for Jin manifestation. The more focused your mind is, the stronger the Qi can be led. When this Qi is used to energize the physical body, the action will be strong. This is the basic theory of internal martial arts. During this mind-Jin manifestation process, the breathing is considered to be a strategy. The breath follows the action, but should be harmonious. When the action is fast, the breathing is fast, and when the action is slow, the breathing is slow. However, at all times, the breathing is deep, harmonious and calm, not shallow and excited. When your breathing becomes excited, your mind will be scattered and confused, and your body will be mal-nourished for oxygen. If your breathing is har-monious, the mind can remain calm, even if your movements and breathing are fast.

13. Once the Yi moves, the shape follows, the posture (is manifested) completely, and the Yi is continuous.

As explained previously, in any action, the Yi (i.e., wisdom mind) is generated first, and the Qi is then led through the physical body for action. Therefore, the mind is always the initiator of any action. However, this mind must be aware of and respond to your part-ner's intention. There must be no division within the mind, no second guessing of deci-sion and action. To do so creates interruptions and breaks in both your intention and the energy it leads through your body for action. However, once the Jin is completely manifest-ed, it will again depend on your mind to give it a new manifestation. The Jin itself can thus be broken, but the Yi must be continued from one action to the next.

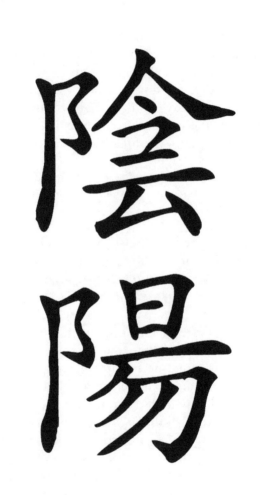

5. Song of Eight Words[13]
Anonymous

Peng (Wardoff), Lu (Rollback), Ji (Press), and
  An (Push) are rare in this world.
Ten martial artists, ten don't know.
If able to be light and agile, also strong and
  hard, (then you gain) Adhere-Connect, Stick-
  Follow with no doubt.
Cai (Pluck), Lie (Split), Zhou (Elbow), and
  Kao (Bump) are even more remarkable.
When used, no need to bother your mind.
If you gain the secret of the words Adhere-
  Connect, Stick-Follow,
Then you will be in the ring and not scattered.

Wardoff, Rollback, Press, and Push are the four basic movements of Taijiquan. Few people understand them properly. The movements are done with Qi-supported Jin, which allows the power to be either soft or hard. One must avoid external muscular power, called Li, which makes movement stiff, clumsy, and stagnant. You must stay light and agile, avoid meeting force with force (i.e., double weighting), and wait for the right opportunity. If you do the right move at the right time in the proper direction, then your techniques will be powerful.

The eight postures are the eight basic fighting Jin patterns of the art, and can be assigned directions according to where your partner's force is moved. Peng (Wardoff) rebounds your partner back in the direction he came from. Lu (Rollback) leads him further than he intended to go in the direction he was attacking. Lie (Split) and Kao (Bump) lead him forward and deflect him slightly sideward. Cai (Pluck) and Zhou (Elbow) can be done so as to catch your partner just as he is starting forward, and strike or unbalance him diagonally to his rear. Ji (Press) and An (Push) deflect your partner and attack at right angles to his motion.

You must also learn "Adhere-Connect, Stick-Follow." This is the technique of remaining lightly attached to your partner, and following him without break or letting up, but also without resistance or force. This is the only way you can really learn how to take advantage of your partner's actions. If you master the first four moves, then the second four will come much more easily, and in time you can do them automatically. But again, your actions must be based on your partner's movements and postures, and this can only come about through "Adhere-Connect, Stick-Follow."

This kind of Jin is developed initially on the hands and the forearms, but once you develop a feeling for it, you can develop the same sensitivity and responsiveness in every part of your body. After a long period of training, if any part of your body is attacked, that part will automatically move just enough to avoid the attack, but not enough to break contact. Just as you move away to evade the attack, you will tend to move forward as your partner withdraws. You need not remain connected to your partner with the same part of your body to utilize this Jin—once the attack is intercepted, For example, the connection can flow from one forearm to the other, and then up to a your shoulder as you perhaps counter with diagonal flying, all without breaking the Jin. This Jin is very subtle, and usually can only be taught in person by a qualified master. The student must feel the Jin in order to fully appreciate its nature.

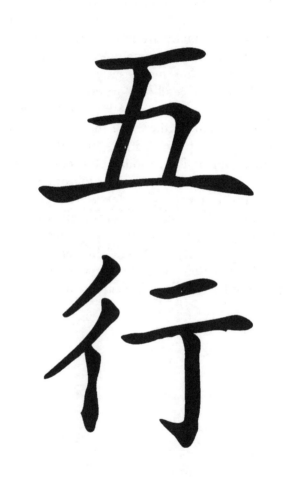

6. Three Important Theses of Taijiquan

Anonymous

A. The Thesis of the Mind Comprehending[1,3]

The waist and the spine are the first masters.
The throat is the second master.
The heart (mind) is the third master.
The (Lower) Dan Tian is the first chancellor.
The fingers and palms are the second chancellors.
The foot and sole are the third chancellors.

In Taijiquan applications, the waist directs all movement, like the steering wheel of a car. In addition, the Jin stored in the correct posture of the spine (i.e., bow), and the Qi from within the spine strengthens the Jin. Without the waist, Jin storage in the torso, and Qi from the spine, you are missing the major center of control, and the major source of power. Therefore, the waist and the spine (i.e., torso) are the first masters.

Even when you have control, and Qi from the spine, if you can't use the Qi, then your efforts are in vain. In order to move Qi to the extremities, the Spirit of Vitality must be raised by coordinating your breathing (exhalation when attacking, inhalation when yielding), and making the Hen-Ha sound in correspondence with the Yin or Yang of the force used. The Hen sound while inhaling is Yin, which builds the Qi in the bone marrow and the Lower Dan Tian. The Ha sound while exhaling is Yang, which leads the Qi to the extremities and beyond the skin for Jin manifestation. When applying these two sounds correctly, the spirit can be condensed and raised, and the Qi can be instantly guided to the extremities for application. Therefore, the throat (breathing and sound) is the second master.

Even when applying the above two principles, the emotional mind (Xin) must be controlled by the wisdom mind. When the emotional mind is excited, although the spirit can be high, the will is scattered and confused. Yet if the emotional mind is completely controlled, then the fighting spirit will be low. The best fighting spirit is raised yet controlled. When you are in this state, your judgment will be clear and accurate, and your spirit will be alert and energized. Thus, the mind (i.e., both emotional and wisdom) is the third master.

The above three factors are important for Taijiquan. However, they are not enough to make the techniques perfect. Unless the Qi is generated from the Lower Dan Tian, it will be weak. It is said "Qi sinks to the Dan Tian." This must be done to keep generating Qi, as well as to increase downward stability.

In addition, you need sensitivity in the fingers and palms to listen to and understand your partner's Jin. This enables you to neutralize and react appropriately.

Finally, if you have mastered all of the above elements but do not have a firm root, then your postures will not be stable, and your Jin will lose its foundation. Therefore, the Lower Dan Tian, the fingers and palms, and the feet and soles are the three chancellors of all Taijiquan techniques.

B. The Marvelous Application of the Entire Body[1]

(You) want your heart (Xin, i.e., emotional mind) to be natural,
And your Yi (i.e., clear thinking or wisdom mind) to be calm,
Then naturally everywhere will be light and agile.

The mastery of the mind over the body is emphasized. Your awareness and perception of things around you must be clear and not distorted by emotions or preconceptions.

(You) want the entire body's Qi to circulate smoothly, (it) must be continuous and non-stop.

Good Qi circulation throughout the body is necessary for Taijiquan and for health. Since Qi is linked with awareness and sensing, good Qi circulation is also necessary for the body to be obedient to the mind.

(You) don't ever want to give up your throat (voice); question every talented person in heaven and earth.

The voice here refers first to the Hen and Ha sounds made during practice, which help to condense the Qi to bone marrow (Hen) and raise the Spirit of Vitality (Ha), and to control and direct energy. Second, you must be humble enough to use your voice to ask guidance of those who have achieved higher levels of ability. There is so much to life and the martial arts that other people's views and experiences are necessary to fill out our own partial understanding. You should always remember, the taller the bamboo grows, the lower it bows. Therefore, you should always be humble, and politely ask questions whenever you can.

If (you are) asked: how can one attain this great achievement, (the answer is) outside and inside,

Fine and coarse, nothing must not be touched upon.

You can specialize in one small area of the art and become very good at it, but the only way to achieve real mastery and true understanding is to explore every facet of the art, which includes the postures on the outside and the Qi on the inside. Large and small, fine and coarse, all aspects must be explored.

C. Seventeen Key Theses[1,3]

1. Rotate on the feet.

The root of your body is in your feet. When your body twists and turns, the movement starts in your feet, and goes all the way up to your fingers and your head. Your root must be stable in order for you to have controlled and accurate motion.

2. Move on the legs.

The legs generate energy. When you walk, your upper body does very little, and the legs do all the work. When you push or yield, your legs move your upper half, which remains relaxed.

3. Spring on the knees.

Your bent knees provide springiness to your legs, which is crucial to the generation and accumulation of Jin. The strength and flexibility of the sinews in the knees determines to a great extent the strength and effectiveness of the whole body.

4. Lively waist.

The waist controls your energy and actions in both offense and defense. Your waist must be flexible and relaxed in order to do this effectively.

5. Agility (Ling) passes through the back.

The energy that is generated by the legs and directed by the waist then passes through the body. The body, especially the back, must be relaxed in order for the energy to move freely and accurately.

6. Shen (Spirit) threads up through the head.

The *Taijiquan Classic* by Wang, Zong-Yue states that an insubstantial energy should lead the head upward, so that it feels as if it were suspended by a thread from above. This helps the rest of the body to relax, and the Spirit of Vitality to rise to the top of the head.

7. *Qi should flow and move (in your entire body).*

Cultivate your Qi so that it fills your whole body and circulates through all the channels. This will clear up stagnant Qi that can cause health problems. Doing the Taijiquan sequence stimulates and moves the Qi, and trains it so that it can support Jin.

8. *Transport (Qi) to the palms.*

To use Taijiquan you have to be able to use the mind to transport Qi instantly to any part of the body, particularly to the hands.

9. *(It) passes into the fingers.*

You must be able to move Qi from your palms into your fingers, for that is where your will expresses itself.

10. *(Qi) condenses into the marrow.*

This is a Yin aspect Jin which stores the Qi in the bone marrow. After many years of practice, the bone becomes very strong. Bone marrow is a factory for producing blood cells. When Qi in the bone marrow is abundant, the blood cells produced will be healthy and abundant, increasing your energy level and maintaining your youth.

11. Approach (the opponent's) Shen (Spirit).

After practicing for a long time, you can reach a level of enlightenment, where you can sense your partner's intentions and Spirit. Then, at your partner's slightest move, you can move first. This phrase can also be translated as: Approach (your) Shen. The highest level of Taijiquan practice is to regulate the spirit. If you can reach such a high level of spiritual enlightenment, then fighting will become meaningless. You will be able to achieve a strategy of fighting without fighting.

12. Concentrate on the ears.

In pushing hands and sparring, you must pay careful attention to your partner. You must be very sensitive to his motion and energy. This is done through the sensitivity of the skin, and also by the eyes. In Taijiquan, this is called "listening."

13. Breathe through the nose.

Breathing, which is normally through the nose, should be regular, relaxed, and natural. Unless you are manifesting Jin with the Ha sound, you should usually keep your mouth closed.

14. Exhale and inhale in the lungs.

This means your breathing should be deep, and begin at the lower abdomen, so that the Qi can sink to the Lower Dan Tian. If you can breathe fully and calmly, your mind will become clear, your Qi will settle, and impurities will be cleansed from your system.

15. To and from the mouth.

This refers to the Hen-Ha sounds made as you draw your partner in, and then expel him.

16. Let the body return to its original state.

After long years of practice, your body will regain the qualities of a baby, and you can respond to everything around you with the simplicity and naturalness of a child.

17. The entire body emits on the hair.

If your entire body is filled with Qi, and all the small channels out to the skin (roots of the hair) are opened, then you will be more sensitive. You can develop your sensing Jins to a very high level, and you can emit Jin from anywhere in your body.

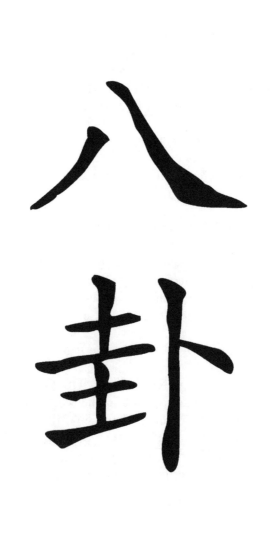

7. The Five Mental Keys to Diligent Study[2]
Anonymous

1. *Study wide and deep.*
2. *Investigate, ask.*
3. *Ponder carefully.*
4. *Clearly discriminate.*
5. *Work perseveringly.*

Taijiquan has been developed and refined over many centuries. To truly master the art, you must study the solo form, including the applications for all the moves, the two-person sequence, weapons, meditation, and Qigong. You should push hands with as many people as possible to experience a wide range of body types and temperaments. You must be humble and open to learning from anyone. The more you ask and investigate, the more you will learn. You must carefully ponder everything you hear and see, discriminating good points from bad, evaluating what is true and false, and determining when something is valid or usable and when it is not. Most important of all is to persevere. It is desirable to have good teachers and helpful to have natural talent, but unless you are willing and able to train diligently, it is all to no avail.

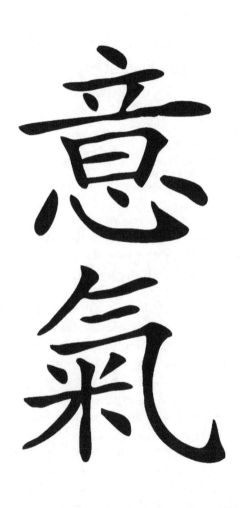

8. Song of Pushing Hands[1-5]
Anonymous

*Be conscientious about Peng (Wardoff), Lu
(Rollback), Ji (Press), and An (Push).
Up and down follow each other, (then) the
opponent (will find it) difficult to enter.*

Wardoff, Rollback, Press, and Push are the
four basic moves of Taiji pushing hands. You
must be serious in your study, and must practice and research these moves extensively to
find out just what they are, and how and when
they are used. When practicing, you and your
partner should adhere lightly to each other,
following the motion back and forth, up and
down. Also, remember that when you attack
high, you are vulnerable and must cover low,
and vice versa. These four postures are like
fundamental building blocks of the art. By
understanding these postures not just as
mechanical movements of the body, but
rather as sign posts to deeper comprehension
of the fundamental energies of the universe,
your Taiji practice can provide you with a
much greater appreciation of the dynamics of
your day to day environment.

Similarly, when your partner attacks high, counterattack low. If you do this, it will be difficult for your partner to get in on you.

No matter (if) he uses enormous power to attack me, (I) use four ounces to lead (him aside), deflecting (his) one thousand pounds.

Taijiquan is based on the principle of not meeting force with force. When a partner attacks with great strength, you lead his attack away from you. The key word here is "lead." You cannot push a large bull around, but if it has a ring through its sensitive nose, you can lead it this way or that with very little force. When a punch is coming at you with great force, you should adhere lightly to it, and lead it slightly off its course. If you try to make a sudden, major change in the course of an incoming attack, you might get bowled over by the forward momentum. Even if you succeeded, you would need to expend considerable force.

Guide (his power) into emptiness, then immediately attack; Adhere-Connect, Stick-Follow, do not lose him.

Your partner expects his attack to meet resistance. If instead, you lead his attack past you, he will lose balance in the direction of his motion. This is the time to attack. Adhere-Connect means to attach a hand to him, and to become one with his motion, wherever he moves. Stick-Follow means to stay with him and not let him get away. Using these techniques, you can overcome hardness with softness.

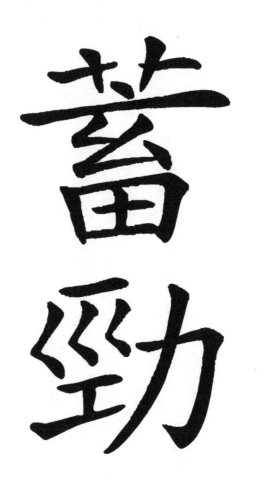

蓄勁

9. Song of the Real Meaning[1]
Anonymous

No shape, no shadow.
Entire body transparent and empty.
Forget (your) surroundings and be natural.
Like a stone chime suspended from West
    Mountain.
Tigers roaring, monkeys screeching.
Clear fountain, peaceful water.
Turbulent river, stormy ocean.
With (your) whole being, develop (your) life.

When practicing Taijiquan you must let go of everything. Your mind must be clear and centered. No concepts (preconceptions) should cloud your vision, no thoughts should hinder your action. The body must be relaxed and stable, so that you can be light and agile. Let go of all thoughts of the past and the future, and be present in the moment. Your body and mind become shapeless, not in that they become amorphous, but in that they become pure potential, casting no shadow in the physical world because your intention has yet to come into being. In this way your body can become in a way transparent to all external forces. Forget your surroundings and just

59

do what needs to be done. Use your breathing as a road to travel into your body and mind — your breath connects the inner and outer worlds.

West Mountain is a famous mountain. "Like a stone chime suspended from West Mountain" means your mind must be clear, your head held as if suspended from above, and your body as stable and rooted as a great mountain. Your root should be both deep and wide, like a mountain's roots, descending into the crust of the earth, supporting your spirit as it reaches higher and higher, like a mountain's peak. The tailbone should be tucked under at all times, allowing you to open your Lumbar spine and connect to your legs. The head should lift up out of your shoulders, with the chin tucked in very slightly in order to gently stretch the cervical spine. Be careful not to thrust the chin forward, creating tension in the lower part of the neck.

Sound is important in Taijiquan, because it is linked to your Qi and the emission of power. Your sound must be as powerful as a tiger's roar and as penetrating as a monkey's screech. If you lift your Spirit (Shen) and guide your Qi throughout your body, your mind will be as clear and pure as a fountain full of spring water. If you practice Taijiquan for a long time, cultivating your Qi, your Qi will fill your body and circulate peacefully.

But, like water, it can move powerfully and quickly so that nothing can stand before it.

This is not something that can be done lightly or casually, for it takes your full attention and effort. When practiced in such a deep and profound way, Taijiquan fills your whole life, tying in to everything else you do. At this stage, the separation between your life and your art disappears, and your efforts are directed at improving yourself as a whole, unified person.

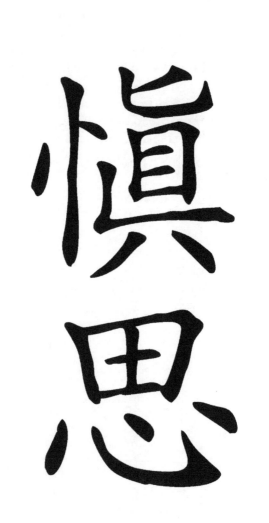

10. Taijiquan Fundamental Key Points[1]

Anonymous

1. An insubstantial energy leads the head (upward).

The head should feel like it is suspended from above. This will raise the Spirit of Vitality and let the whole body move lightly and agilely.

2. The eye gazes with concentrated Spirit.

When a person has concentrated and raised his Spirit, his eyes will be bright and he can pay attention to even the slightest movement of his partner.

3. Hold the chest in, arc the back.

The back between the shoulders has the feeling of being lifted, and the chest is slightly sunken. This lets the chest relax and creates a defensive circle using your back and arms. This is also used to neutralize your partner's attack and to store energy within the posture. This is the key to Peng (Wardoff) Jin.

4. Sink the shoulders, drop the elbows.

Dropping the shoulders and elbows helps relaxation, and facilitates the transmission of energy into the hands. When the elbows and shoulders are sunk, the Jin can thread through from the waist to the hands, so that they can function as one unit. Otherwise, the Jin will be broken. Furthermore, sinking the elbows and shoulders will seal major cavities, such as the armpits, against attack. This posture also helps you neutralize attacks, because your body is compact, and can more easily evade or deflect an attack.

5. Settle the wrists, extend the fingers.

When the hand is extended palm downward, to "settle the wrist" means to drop the wrist slightly, so that the base of the palm is facing forward. This facilitates striking with the palm. Remember to keep the wrist relaxed. "Extend the fingers" means to let the fingers be straight, but not tensed. This should not be forced. Gradually get used to holding the fingers fairly straight, so that there is no hindrance to the flow of blood and Qi. This is the key to Push (An) Jin.

6. Body central and upright.

The body should be straight and erect, not leaning to any side.

7. *Pull up the tailbone.*

The tailbone should be pulled slightly in and up, in order to keep the pelvis at the proper angle and the lower back straight. When the tip of the tailbone is allowed to move backward, the pelvis tilts forward, and the lower back curves inward. This deprives the lower abdomen of its support, and lets the belly bulge forward. A curved lower back also hinders the efficient transmission of energy up and down the spine. Therefore, it is very important to keep the tailbone tucked in and under.

8. *Relax (your) waist and relax (your) thighs.*

The waist controls and directs the application of force. The thighs connect the waist to the knees, which are very important to all movement, and in the generation of force by the legs. It is therefore important to keep the waist and thighs relaxed and movable.

9. *The knees look relaxed, but are not relaxed.*

In Taijiquan, the Jin is generated from the legs. In order to do this, the legs must behave like springs to release the power. Therefore, the knees must be relaxed. However, the legs are also vital for strategic stepping during a fight, so they must move swiftly yet remain firm. In order to move fast with a firm root, the knees must be able to vary their tension skillfully. This sentence means that the knees look relaxed, but can be tensed whenever necessary.

10. *Soles touch the ground. (Feet flat on the ground.)*

The feet (or foot) must always be flat on the ground and relaxed, so that your root will be stable. Unless a specific posture calls for it, don't rest your weight on just the heels or the toes, but instead let the weight spread over the whole of the foot. Be careful not to let the inner arches and ankles collapse. Keep your attention on the center of the foot, a little bit behind the Bubbling Well point. This is where the center of gravity naturally falls.

11. *Top and bottom follow each other, the entire body should be united as one (i.e., coordinate harmoniously).*

The entire body must move in a unified, coordinated way. Your upper body movement determines what your legs do, and your legs control your upper body. Your arms and legs must move together.

12. Distinguish insubstantial and substantial.

The body, both as a whole and in each of its parts, has a substantial and an insubstantial aspect. Usually, only one leg and one arm should be substantial at any time. What parts of the body are either substantial or insubstantial depends upon your partner's actions. When your partner is substantial, you become insubstantial where he contacts you, and substantial somewhere else, either left or right, up or down. Also, you must clearly judge whether your partner's attack is substantial or insubstantial. Very often, a person can change a substantial force into an insubstantial one, and vice versa. Therefore, you must know your Yin and Yang, and also your partner's Yin and Yang. Then you know your partner, but your partner doesn't know you. You can control him, but you cannot be controlled.

13. Internal and external are mutually coordinated. Breathe naturally.

Breathing, Qi, muscular strength and Yi must all act together. Breathing should be relaxed, and should match your actions in a comfortable way. If the breathing is tense or jerky, then there is tension in the body, the mind is not still, and the Qi flow is hindered and unable to support the Jin.

14. Use Yi (mind), not Li (strength).

This means you should use skill, technique, and intelligence to defeat your partner, and not just overwhelm him with strength. It also means that when you do a technique, you should think only of what you are doing—e.g., pushing your partner, locking an arm, etc. Do not think of Qi, strength, or your body, for this will split your attention and will weaken the technique. When you use your Yi (mind) to move, the Qi is automatically circulated, but when you use Li, you will be more tense and the Qi circulation will be hindered.

15. Qi circulates through the whole body; dividing, it moves up and down.

In Taijiquan, the Qi must not only be abundant, it must also circulate smoothly through the entire body. If the Qi can circulate freely, then the mind can lead the Qi to energize muscular power for efficient Jin manifestation. When you are leading the Qi for Jin manifestation, the Qi is divided into two major flows, one through the spine, manifested at the fingers, and the other down to the bottom of the feet, to build up a firm root. It is said: "There is an up, there is a down, there is a forward, there is a backward." This means that you are centered.

16. Yi and Qi mutually linked (i.e., Yi moves, Qi follows).

Qi follows the mind, so that wherever you put your attention, Qi accumulates. This is the reason that mental self-discipline is so important.

17. Every form of every posture follows smoothly; no forcing, no opposition, the entire body is comfortable.

The entire sequence should flow smoothly, from beginning to end. There should be no breaks, jerks, or sharp angles. The movements should be natural and comfortable for your body. In each posture, every part of the body contributes, either directly or by counterbalancing. No part of the body should hinder this unified flow.

18. Each form smooth.

Every form in the sequence should be done smoothly, with Yi, Qi, and the body all unified.

19. Postures should not be too little or too much (i.e., neither insufficient nor excessive). (The postures) should seek to be centered and upright.

Your body should be natural, centered, balanced, and controlled. Your arms and legs should neither be too extended nor drawn in too much. Strive to be efficient.

20. *Your applications should be concealed, and not exposed.*

Your partner should not be able to sense or predict your intentions. Your attack and defense should be concealed and unpredictable, in order to confuse your partner.

21. *Attain stillness in motion.*

You should maintain a meditative state while moving, then you will be calm and your mind clear.

22. *Attain motion in stillness.*

If you are in a meditative state you will move your Qi and body naturally and correctly without conscious effort.

23. *Light, then agile; agile, then move; move, then vary.*

This is Taijiquan in a nutshell. The first requirement is to clear the mind, relax the body, and circulate the Qi. Then you will be light. If you adhere to your partner, not resisting and not letting go, then you will be agile. You can then move to attack and defend, but remember to vary your techniques so that your intentions cannot be read by your partner.

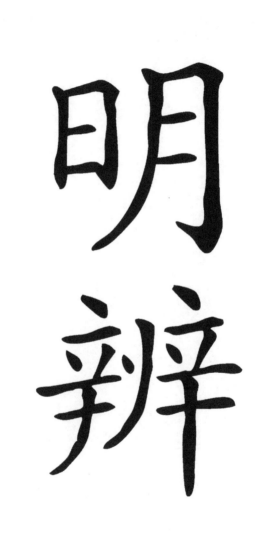

11. Song of Application[13]
Anonymous

*Light, agile, and alive, seek Dong Jin
    (Understanding Jin);*
*Yin and Yang cooperate mutually without the
    fault of stagnation;*
*If (you) acquire (the trick), four ounces neutral-
    izes one thousand pounds;*
*Expand and close, stimulate the "drum," the
    center will be steady.*

"Alive" here means alert and active. In practice you must pay close attention to your partner.
In time, you can interpret his intention from the
slightest of motions (i.e., understanding Jin).
Where your partner is heavy, you are light.
When one part of you is light, another part of
you is heavy. You and your partner continually
follow one another, never resisting, never sepa-
rating. In this way the motion will continue to
flow. In time you will acquire the knack of being
light enough to avoid your partner's attack, and
substantial and controlled enough to deflect or
attack him. Your postures alternately open and
close with the circumstances. The drum is the
abdomen, in the area of the Lower Dan Tian.
You stimulate the Qi centered there with sound,

attention, breathing and movement. This strengthens the Qi and exercises your control of it. When your attention and actions are thus centered on the Lower Dan Tian, your stance will be stable, and your mind calm and clear.

12. Old Taijiquan Classic of Qing Qian Long Dynasty[*1]

Anonymous

*Follow the neck to thread (the Qi) to the head,
the two shoulders relaxed.*
*Condense the strong lower Qi, and support the
crotch (hips).*
*The stomach sound extends the Jin to strength-
en the two fists' (Jin).*
*Five toes grasp the ground, the top bent like a
bow.*

An insubstantial energy lifts the head and straightens the neck. This allows the Qi to flow naturally, and keeps the shoulders relaxed and sunk. The Qi is condensed into the Lower Dan Tian. The Qi is led to the feet to build up a firm root, and at the same time there is force coming up and supporting the hips. This sinking and lifting allows the posture to be stable and flexible. When this happens, the Qi can also be led upward to the arms for Jin manifestation.

Be sure to draw back in following manifestation of an offensive Jin. This helps to sharpen the Jin's penetrating power, and helps to maintain your stability.

*1736-1796 A.D.

The Ha sound, which comes from the "stomach" or abdomen, helps you raise the Spirit of Vitality, coordinate Qi and Jin, and extend energy out to your hands. It should be uttered with a loud, sharp vocalization from the diaphragm. Be careful not to vocalize the "Ha" sound from the throat, since this will not help you manifest power, and can cause injury to your voice.

When your feet "grasp the ground," the root should be firm and alive, but should still remain relaxed. Imagine that you can actually sink yourself down into the ground using the Bubbling Well cavities. The legs should be bent like a bow. They should neither be completely straight, nor should the knee of the front leg be bent past a forty-five degree angle.

> Move lightly and with agility and condense the
>   Spirit internally.
> Don't be broken and then continuous, refine
>   your one Qi.
> Left and right as appropriate have insubstantial
>   and substantial places.
> When Yi (mind) is up, this implies down; and
>   return post-birth (Qi to pre-birth state).

You should be light and agile and should keep your Spirit inside. If you expose your Spirit externally, people can see what you are doing and thinking. By keeping your Spirit internal, you can hide your intention until the time is right. Your postures and motion should be fluid and continuous, and all should be one flow of Qi. The different parts of the body are substantial or insubstantial, and this changes constantly with the circumstances. To do this appropriately requires correct timing.

When your attention is up, don't forget down. When your partner attacks down, don't forget up. All of this is not done with post-birth strength (Li), but rather with Qi-supported Jin. Therefore, you should learn how to return the post-birth Qi to its original state (i.e., pre-birth state). Post-Birth Qi comes from the food we eat and the air we breath. Pre-Birth Qi was given to us with the genetic material we inherited from our parents. In this way, the Pre-Birth Qi is more pure, being closer in source to the creative energy of the universe. Pre-Birth Qi is produced and stored in the Lower Dan Tian. You should endeavour to support your Jin with this type of Qi, rather than the local Qi in the limbs.

> Grasp and hold the Dan Tian to train internal Gongfu. Hen, Ha, two Qi's are marvelous and infinite.
> Move open, calm close, bend and extend following (your opponent).
> Slow respond (slow), fast follow (fast), the principles must be understood thoroughly.

When your attention remains on your Lower Dan Tian, you will gradually generate internal energy. When you coordinate this with your breathing and motions, your Gongfu will be internal and superior to the external variety. The two sounds, Hen and Ha, help you to mobilize and express your energy. When you move, you open or extend your energy. When you close, you accumulate energy, but calmly, so your partner doesn't notice.

You bend and extend, contract and expand, yield and adhere, neutralize and attack, all depending upon your partner. You move slow or fast, following your partner, and always according to the Taiji principles.

> *Suddenly disappear, suddenly appear. Forward,*
>   *then expand.*
> *A feather cannot be added; be perfect like the*
>   *Daoist bible.*
> *Hand slow, hand fast, all not alike.*
> *Four ounces repel a thousand pounds,*
> *apply this principle and neutralize well.*

As you exchange substantial and insubstantial, you disappear in front of your partner's attack and reappear elsewhere to attack him. You remain insubstantial, and when you find an opportunity you move forward and "expand," i.e., become substantial. This is just like the Taiji diagram, where each side is small where the other side is large, and large where the other side is small. You must be so light, agile, and responsive that a feather cannot touch you without setting you in motion. If you can do this, your art will be as perfect as the Daoist bible.

Slow or fast, the situation is always changing, but if you adhere to the principles, you can neutralize an attack of a thousand pounds with four ounces.

> *Peng (Wardoff), Lu (Rollback), Ji (Press), An (Push) are the four main directions.*
> *Cai (Pluck), Lie (Split), Zhou (Elbow), Kao (Bump) complete the four diagonal corners.*
> *Qian (Heaven), Kun (Earth), Zhen (Thunder), Dui (Lake) are the eight trigrams.*
> *Forward, backward, look to the left, look to the right, and central equilibrium are the five elements*

Taijiquan is said to be comprised of thirteen postures. There are the eight basic moves and the five directions. These are coordinated with the eight trigrams (the author of this article lists only four of the eight trigrams, assuming the reader is already quite familiar with them) and the five elements.

Qian (Heaven)	Peng (Wardoff)
Kun (Earth)	Lu (Rollback)
Kan (Water)	Ji (Press)
Li (Fire)	An (Push)

Xun (Wind)	Cai (Pluck)
Zhen (Thunder)	Lie (Split)
Dui (Lake)	Zhou (Elbow)
Gen (Mountain)	Kao (Bump)

Jin Bu (Forward)	Jin (Metal)
Tui Bu (Backward)	Mu (Wood)
Zuo Gu (Left)	Shui (Water)
You Pan (Right)	Huo (Fire)
Zhong Ding (Center)	Tu (Earth)

Extremely soft means hardness. That means extremely insubstantial and agile.

When you transport (Qi) it is like drawing silk from a cocoon.

Everywhere clear. Open and expanding, tight and compact, one right after the other, should be threaded together tightly.

Wait for the opportunity, then move as a cat moves.

In Taijiquan, you achieve hardness through softness. You remain light and agile, avoiding your partner's attack, and waiting for the opportunity when you can mobilize all your forces and attack with certainty. When you are experienced at moving Qi throughout your body, you can clearly sense the location and path of the energy.

When you are opening and closing, expanding and contracting in response to your partner's moves, your postures should mesh together seamlessly, so that there is no opportunity for him to attack. You adhere and stick, neutralize and follow, always paying careful attention. When the opportunity to attack presents itself, you attack instantly.

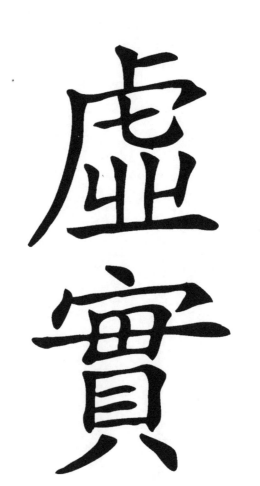

虛實

13. Song of Comprehension and Application[7]
Anonymous

*Taijiquan, thirteen postures, it's marvelous,
(because there are) two Qi's, discriminated as
Yin and Yang.*

Because it includes eight basic movements and five steppings in its fighting strategy, Taijiquan is also called the thirteen postures. Other names for Taijiquan include Soft Sequence (Mian Quan), and Long Sequence (Chang Quan). This extraordinary training and fighting strategy is made up of two Qi's—Yin and Yang. All the movements, breathing, Qi circulation, and techniques are based on Yin and Yang principles, and derive into insubstantial and substantial fighting strategies.

*(From Yin and Yang, it) derives and generates a
thousand million (techniques), all belonging
to one (principle).
All belongs to one. Taijiquan has two poles,
four phases, it is infinite.*

From Yin and Yang (insubstantial and substantial) fighting strategies, the principle of neutralization is generated. From the principle of neutralization, numerous techniques are created. Though the techniques are many, there is only one principle.

Taiji's two poles—Yin and Yang—generate four phases; the four phases generate eight trigrams, the eight trigrams generate sixty-four hexagrams, and the hexagrams generate everything else. The four phases are extreme Yin, extreme Yang, deficient Yin and deficient Yang.

The Chinese translated here as "infinite" is literally "blurred no sides." This has the feeling of being on a foggy river where everything is indistinct and the shores cannot be seen. This concept of infinity is one of formlessness and eternal, inexhaustible potential, rather than pure spatial vastness, as with the physical universe, or of endless iteration, as with mathematical infinities.

> (If you) follow the wind, how can your head be
>   suspended? I have one guiding sentence.
> Today I want to tell it to the people who can
>   comprehend.
> (If) the Bubbling Well (Yongquan cavity) has
>   no root, the waist has no master,
> (Then) you can try hard to learn until you
>   almost die, you will still not succeed.

If you sway and move around like a kite in the wind, you cannot cultivate the feeling of being suspended from above. You must keep

the body straight and erect, with an insubstantial energy lifting the head and giving
you the feeling of being suspended from
above. At the same time, you must sink your
Qi to the soles of the feet into the Bubbling
Well cavities.

Having a good root is absolutely essential
for getting force out to the hands, or to any
part of the body, for any of the techniques. A
good root is also necessary for effective use of
the waist. If there is no root and waist control,
all of your practice is in vain, and your techniques are useless. Proper rooting incorpo-
rates centering, balancing, and correct
stance. Each of these elements must be
trained to the point of habit in order to enable
you to find your root under all possible circumstances. The single most common error
made by Taiji martial artists—and martial
artists in general—is the loss of root, and the
rising of the center, during stressful situa-
tions.

*When comprehension and application mutually
support one another—is there any other trick
to do this?*
*(No), because marvelous Qi can approach the
hands.*

A Taijiquan practitioner must learn the
principles and techniques first, and then he
should ponder and comprehend the deeper

meaning of the theory. Only after that can he apply all the theory and techniques. After he has gained enough experience in applying the techniques, he should go back to the theory and ponder again, and then apply it to the techniques and so on. Comprehension and application mutually support each other, and will help one become a high level Taiji artist. If one practices this way, his Qi can reach his hands. This will not only benefit his health, but will also be useful in martial applications.

> Peng (Wardoff), Lu (Rollback), Ji (Press), An (Push),
> Cai (Pluck), Lie (Split), Zhou (Elbow), Kao (Bump),
> and Jin (Forward), Tui (Backward), Gu (Left), Pan (Right), and Ding (Center).
> Don't neutralize, automatically neutralize; (don't) yield, automatically yield.

For all thirteen postures, one should follow the rule of natural response. Yielding and neutralizing should not be big, conscious moves. They should be natural and automatic. Don't try to yield. Stay calm and centered and let it happen automatically. Just stick to your partner, follow, and automatically neutralize.

> (When you) wish the foot to go forward, (you) must push off from the rear (foot).
> (Your) body is like moving clouds. (When you)

strike with the hands, why use hands?
The entire body is hands, but the hands are not
(your) hands.
However (you) must be careful to protect what
should be protected at all times.

When you wish to move, push off the rear foot. Move lightly like a cloud. When you strike, don't use the force of the arms. Instead, use the force of the whole body, generated from the legs and controlled by the waist. It may not be necessary to use the hands at all. Instead, you may use any part of the body in contact with your partner. However, when you do this you must remember to do whatever is necessary to protect yourself.

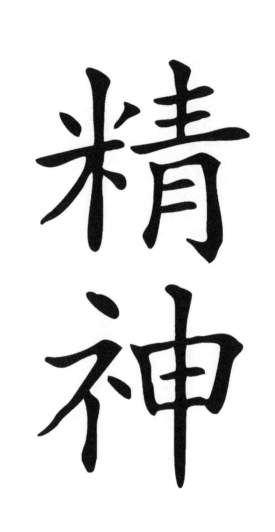

14. Song of the Thirteen Postures[1,4,5]
Anonymous

*All the thirteen postures (of Taijiquan) must not
be treated lightly. The meaning of life originates at the waist.*

The thirteen postures are the foundation of
Taijiquan. The waist is important because it
governs all of your movements, and because Qi
is generated and stored in the Lower Dan Tian.

*(When you) vary and exchange insubstantial
and substantial (you) must take care that Qi
(circulates) in the entire body without the
slightest stagnation.*

Insubstantial is a Yin strategy, while substantial is a Yang strategy. When you change
these two Yin and Yang strategies, you must
be skillful, active, and alive, and know what
you are doing. In order to reach this stage,
you must be relaxed, responsive, alert, and
have a high Spirit of Vitality. If you can
achieve these conditions, the Qi circulating
in your body will be smooth, and can reach
any place in the body freely and naturally.

*Touch (i.e., feel, sense, or find) the movement in
the stillness, (although there is) stillness even
in movement. Vary (your) response to the
opponent and show the marvelous techniques.*

To touch means to feel, to sense, to detect,
to direct, or to govern. Feeling is the language
which links the mind and the body. If you can
build up a high degree of sensitivity, your
mind can respond and govern the body's
movement skillfully.

Taiji has been called meditation in
motion. While moving, the mind is still, centered and quiet, as in sitting meditation. At
the same time, while in this meditative state,
one is still actively circulating Qi. When
attacked, remain in the meditative state, calm
and aware. When the principles have been
learned and internalized, you can respond
naturally and comfortably to your partner's
moves. Taiji is the art of change. As you follow your partner's actions, your response sub-
tly changes and varies with the situation.

*Pay attention to every posture and gauge its
purpose, (then you will) gain (the art) without wasting your time and energy.*

The care and seriousness you put into your
study determines the degrees of success you
will have. Every posture has its nature, meaning, and purpose, and must be researched and
studied before it can be really understood.

If you can do this, then you will have
gained the essence and the root of each movement. Since all of the Taiji movements and
theory are built upon the Dao, once you have
grasped the keys to pondering and analyzing,
you will soon gain the meaning and the purpose of other postures. However,. if you do
not ponder, analyze, and then practice intel-
ligently, you will remain at a superficial level.

In every movement the heart (mind) remains on
the waist, the abdomen is relaxed and clear,
and Qi rises up.

In all the postures the principle (i.e., the
Dao) is the same: the mind must remain on
the Lower Dan Tian. In Chinese Qigong
practice, it is emphasized that you keep the
mind on the Lower Dan Tian (Yi Shou Dan
Tian). When the mind stays on the Lower
Dan Tian, you will be centered and the Qi
can be raised up to an abundant level. In
order to reach this stage, your abdominal area
must be relaxed, and the mind must be calm
and clear. When this happens, you can use
your mind to lead the Qi (Yi Yi Yin Qi), circulating in the entire body strongly and without stagnation.

The tailbone is central and upright, the Spirit is
threaded through the head. The entire body is
light and easy (relaxed), the top of the head
is suspended.

In order to keep the body centered, and raise up the Spirit of Vitality to a high level, the torso must be upright. To reach this goal, the lower vertebrae must be erect and the back straight. When this happens, the Mingmen (Gv-4)(i.e., life door) on the back (between L2 and L3) will be opened, and this allows the Qi to be led upward, following the spine, and finally spread the Qi to the upper limbs. Keeping the tailbone erect is the crucial key to opening the Mingmen cavity in Grand Qi Circulation Meditation (Da Zhou Tian).

In addition, when your body is centered, you can relax, and the movement can be easy and natural. Under these conditions, if you can raise up the Spirit of Vitality, you can fight against sickness or compete with your partner effectively and efficiently.

Pay attention carefully in (your) research, bent-extended, open-closed follow their freedom.

Bent-extended, open-closed are the tricks of pushing hands. Bend to neutralize your partner's power, at the same time close to store your Jin, and then open and extend to emit your Jin. All these techniques must be natural and freely follow your partner's intention. Then you can Adhere-Connect, Stick-Follow and defeat your partner. If you do not research these tricks with all your heart, you will not gain the key to Taijiquan.

*To enter the door and be led along the way,
(one) needs oral instruction; practice without
ceasing, the way is through self-study.*

To learn Taijiquan well a teacher is needed. There are so many subtleties that it is very easy to get something wrong, or emphasize the wrong things. It is said "a slight error can cause a thousand mile divergence." Traditionally, in the martial arts there were two kinds of students—the outer and the inner. The outer students were often accepted for their money or to test their seriousness. They were taught only the forms and a minimum of applications and principles. Once a student was judged worthy, he was taken into the temple and shown the inner secrets of the style. Today, it is often much easier to learn the secrets of a martial art, because so much has been published. However, having a good teacher in the flesh is still almost a necessity. Once one has been shown the way, the only thing remaining is to practice unceasingly, and to continually research on one's own.

*If asked, what is the standard (criteria) of its
(thirteen postures) application, (the answer
is) Yi (mind) and Qi are the master, and the
bones and muscles are the chancellor.*

The criterion for judging whether the postures are applied correctly is: are the mind and Qi directing the movement? All movement is done with Jin supported by Qi and directed by Yi (mind). If the movement is done only with bones and muscles, it is considered Li, or muscular strength, and is incorrect.

Investigate in detail what the ultimate meaning (i.e., purpose) is: to increase the age, extend the years, and achieve never-aging youthfulness.

You must remember that the ultimate goal of Taijiquan is to maintain a healthy body and a youthful mind.

The song, the song, one hundred and forty (words), every word is real and true, no meaning is left behind. If not approached from this (song), (your) time and energy are wasted in vain, and (you will) sigh in regret.

Whether you study the art for health or self-defense, you must follow the words of this song or your efforts will be wasted.

References

1. 太極拳・刀、劍、桿、散手合編，陳炎林著。

2. 太極拳術，顧留馨著，上海體育出版社，1992。

3. 楊禹廷太極拳系列、秘要集錦，李秉慈、翁福麒編著，奧林匹克出版社，1990。

4. 太極拳全書，人民體育出版社，198 。

5. 太極拳講義，吳公藻編，上海書店，1985。

6. *Lost Tai-Chi Classics from the Late Ch'ing Dynasty*, Douglas Wile, 1996.

7. *Tai Chi Theory & Martial Power*, Dr. Yang, Jwing-Ming, YMAA, 1996.

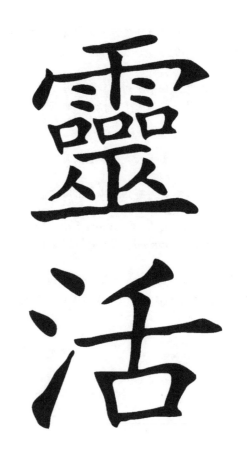

Appendix A
Original Chinese of the Poems and Treatises

1. 太極拳論
張三豐

一舉動，週身俱要輕靈，尤須貫穿。

氣宜鼓盪，神宜內斂。

無使有缺陷處，無使有凸凹處，無使有續斷處。

其根在腳，發於腿，主宰於腰，形於手指。由腳而腿而腰，總須完整一氣。向前退後，乃能得機得勢。

有不得機得勢處，身便散亂。其病必於腰腿求之。

上下前後左右皆然。凡此皆是意，不在外面。

有上即有下，有前即有後，有左即有右。如意要向上，即寓下意。若將物掀起，而加以挫之之意。斯其根自斷，乃壞之速而無疑。

虛實宜分清楚，一處有一處虛實，處處總是如此。周身節節貫串，無令絲毫間斷耳。

長拳者如長江大海滔滔不絕也。

十三勢者，掤、攦、擠、按、採、挒、肘、靠，此八卦也。進步、退步、左顧、右盼、中定，此五行也。掤、攦、擠、按，即乾、坤、坎、離，四正方也。採、挒、肘、靠，即巽、震、兌、艮，四斜角也。進、退、顧、盼、定，即金、木、水、火、土也。合之則爲十三勢也。

2. 太極拳經
王宗岳

太極者，無極而生，動靜之機，陰陽之母也。動之則分，靜之則合。

無過不及，隨曲就伸。

人剛我柔謂之走，我順人背謂之黏。

動急則急應，動緩則緩隨，雖變化萬端，而理為一貫。

由著熟而漸悟懂勁，由懂勁而階及神明。然非用功之久，不能豁然貫通焉。

虛領頂勁，氣沈丹田。

不偏不倚，忽隱忽現。

左重則左虛，右重則右杳。仰之則彌高，俯之則彌深，進之則愈長，退之則愈促，一羽不能加，蠅蟲不能落，人不知我，我獨知人，英雄所向無敵，蓋由此而及也。斯技旁門甚多，雖勢有區別，概不外壯欺弱，慢讓快耳。有力打無力，手慢讓手快。皆是先天自然之能，非關學力而有為也。

查四兩撥千金之句，顯非力勝。觀耄耋能禦眾之形，快何能為。

立如平準，活似車輪。

偏沈則隨，雙重則滯。每見數年純功，不能運化者，率為人制，雙重之病未能悟耳。

欲避此病須知陰陽。粘即是走，走即是粘。陰不離陽，陽不離陰，陰陽相濟，方為懂勁。

懂勁後愈練愈精，默識揣摩，漸至從心所
欲。

本是捨己從人，多誤捨近圖遠。斯謂差之
毫釐，謬以千里，學者不可不詳辨焉。

此論句句切要，並無一字數衍陪襯，非有
夙慧不能悟也。先師不肯妄傳，非獨擇人
，亦恐枉費功夫耳。

3. 四句要言
楊禹廷

關節要鬆，皮毛要攻，節節貫串，虛靈在
中。

4. 調身十三要點
顧留馨

1. 心靜用意，身正體鬆。
2. 由鬆入柔，柔中寓剛。
3. 弧形螺旋，中正體圓。
4. 源動腰脊，勁貫四梢。
5. 三尖六合，上下一線。
6. 虛領頂勁，氣沉丹田。
7. 含胸拔背，落胯塌腰。
8. 垂肩沉肘，坐腕舒指。
9. 屈膝圓襠，骶骨有力。
10. 眼隨手轉，步隨身換。
11. 速度均勻，輕沉兼備。
12. 內動外發，呼吸協調。
13. 意動形隨，勢完意連。

5. 八字歌

拥攦擠按世界稀，十個藝人十不知。
若能輕靈並堅硬，沾連黏隨俱無疑。
採挒肘靠更出奇，行之不用費心思。
果得沾連黏隨字，得其環中不支離。

6. 太極拳之三要論
A. 心會論

腰脊爲第一主宰。
喉頭爲第二主宰。
心地爲第三主宰。
丹田爲第一賓輔。
指掌爲第二賓輔。
足掌爲第三賓輔。

B. 週身大用論

要心性與意靜，自然無處不輕靈。
要遍體氣流行，一定繼續不能停。
要喉頭永不拋，問盡天下眾英豪。
如詢大功因何得，表裡精粗無不到。

C. 十七關要論

1. 旋之於足
2. 行之於腿
3. 縱之於膝
4. 活潑於腰
5. 靈通於背
6. 神貫於頂
7. 流行於氣
8. 運之於掌
9. 通之於指

10. 斂之於髓
11. 達之於神
12. 凝之於耳
13. 息之於鼻
14. 呼吸於肺
15. 往來於口
16. 渾靈於身
17. 全身發之於毛

7. 用功五誌

博學　審問　慎思　明辨　篤行

8. 打手歌

掤攦擠按須認眞，上下相隨人難進。
任他巨力來打我，牽動四兩撥千斤。
引進落空合即出，沾連黏隨不丟頂。

9. 眞義歌

無形無象。　　　全身透空。
忘物自然。　　　西山懸磬。
虎吼猿鳴。　　　泉清水靜。
翻江鬧海。　　　盡性立命。

10. 太極拳基本要點

1. 虛領頂勁。
2. 眼神注視。
3. 含胸拔背。
4. 沈肩垂肘。
5. 坐腕伸指。
6. 身體中正。

7. 尾閭收住。

8. 鬆腰鬆胯。

9. 膝部似鬆非鬆。

10. 足掌貼地。

11. 上下相隨，週身一致。

12. 分清虛實。

13. 內外相合，呼吸自然。

14. 用意不用力。

15. 氣遍週身，分行上下。

16. 意氣相連。

17. 式式勢順，不拗不背，週身舒適。

18. 式式均勻。

19. 姿勢無過或不及，當求其中正。

20. 用法含而不露。

21. 動中求靜。

22. 靜中求動。

23. 輕則靈，靈則動，動則變。

11. 功用歌

輕靈活潑求懂勁，陰陽相濟無滯病，
若得四兩撥千斤，開合鼓盪主宰定。

12. 乾隆舊抄本歌訣

順項貫頂兩膀鬆，束烈下氣把襠撐，
胃音開勁兩捶爭，五指抓地上彎弓。
舉動輕靈神內斂，莫教斷續一氣研，
左宜右有虛實處，意上寓下後天還。
拿住丹田練內功，哼哈二氣妙無窮，
動分靜合屈伸就，緩應急隨理貫通。
忽隱忽現進則長，一羽不加至道藏，
手慢手快皆非似，四兩撥千運化良。

掤攦擠按四方正，採挒肘靠斜角成，
乾坤震兌乃八卦，進退顧盼定五行。
極柔即剛極虛靈，運若抽絲處處明，
開展緊湊乃縝密，待機而動如貓行。

13. 體用歌

太極拳，十三式，妙在二氣分陰陽。化生
千億歸抱一，歸抱一，太極拳兩儀四象渾
無邊。

御風何似頂頭懸，我有一轉語，今爲知者
吐。湧泉無根，腰無主，力學垂死終無捕
。

體用相兼豈有他，浩然氣能行乎手。掤攦
擠按採挒肘，靠及進退顧盼定，不化自化
走自走。

足欲向前先挫後，身似行雲打手安用手，
渾身是手手非手，但須方寸隨時守所守。

14. 十三勢歌

十三總勢莫輕視，命意源頭在腰際。
變換虛實須留意，氣遍身軀不少滯。
靜中觸動動猶靜，應敵變化示神奇。
勢勢存心揆用意，得來全不費功夫。
刻刻留心在腰間，胸腹鬆淨氣騰然。
尾閭中正神貫頂，滿身輕利頂頭懸。
仔細留心向推求，屈伸開合聽自由。
入門引路須口授，功夫無息法自然。
若問體用何爲準，意氣君來骨肉臣。
詳推用意終何在，益壽延年不老春。
歌兮歌兮百四十，字字眞切義無疑。
若不向此推求去，枉費功夫貽歎息。

Appendix B
Translation and Glossary of Chinese Terms

An 按
Push. A technique for pushing or striking the opponent. It is one of the Four Directions of the eight basic Taiji fighting techniques, which correspond to the Eight Trigrams (Bagua).

Ba Men 八門
Eight doors. The eight strategic movements in Taijiquan thirteen postures.

Baihui 百會
Literally, "hundred meeting." An important acupuncture cavity located on the top of the head. The Baihui cavity belongs to the Governing Vessel.

Cai 採
Pluck. A technique for unbalancing the opponent or pulling him into an exposed position. One of the Four Corners of the eight basic Taiji fighting techniques.

Chang Chuan (Changquan) 長拳
Long Fist or Long Sequence. When it means Long Fist, it is a northern Shaolin Chinese martial style which specializes in kicking techniques. When it means Long Sequence, it refers to Taijiquan and implies that the Taiji sequence is long and flowing like a river.

Chang 長
To Grow. Another meaning is "Long."

Cheng, Gin-Gsao 曾金灶
Dr. Yang, Jwing-Ming's White Crane master.

Chin Na (Qin Na) 擒拿
Grasp and Control. An aspect of Chinese martial arts training, Qin Na specializes in controlling the enemy through "misplacing the bone," "dividing the muscle," "sealing the breath," and "cavity press."

Chong 重
Layering. The same character, when pronounced as Zhong, means weight or heaviness.

Da Zhou Tian 大周天
Grand Circulation. A Qigong training method in which the Qi is led to circulate throughout the entire body.

Dan Tian 丹田
Field of Elixir. There are three Dan Tians in the body: the brain, the solar plexus area, and the lower abdomen. Taiji is primarily interested in the Lower Dan Tian. It is considered the reservoir of Qi, and is located approximately one and one-half inches below the navel and about a third of the way toward the spine. In acupuncture this point is known as Qihai (Sea of Qi).

Dao 道
The "way," by implication the "natural way."

Dong Jin 懂勁
Means "understanding Jin." One of the Taiji Jins, through skin listening (i.e., feeling).

Dui 兌
One of the Eight Trigrams (Bagua). Corresponds to Lake.

Gen 艮
One of the eight trigrams (Bagua). Corresponds to Mountain.

Gongfu (Kung Fu) 功夫
Energy and Time. Anything which takes time and energy to master is called Gongfu. In recent times it has come to mean Chinese martial arts.

Gu Dang 鼓盪
Means the drum is full and resounding (due to vibration).

Gu, Liu-Xing 顧留馨
A well known Taijiquan master during the 1950's.

Guoshu (Kuoshu) 國術
National Technique. The name for Chinese martial arts used by Chiang, Kai-Shek since 1926, and still used in Taiwan. Mainland China uses the term Wushu.

Ha 哈
One of the two sounds used in Taijiquan and other Chinese martial styles. The Ha sound is positive (Yang) and is used to raise the Spirit of Vitality, enabling power to reach its maximum.

Haidi 海底
Sea Bottom. The head is the heaven and the perineum is the sea bottom.

Hen 哼
One of the two sounds used in Taijiquan. When done on the inhale, the Hen sound is purely negative (Yin). It condenses the Yi and Qi into the bone marrow. When done on the exhale, Hen is negative with some positive. This allows you to attack while conserving some energy.

Huiyin (Co-1) 會陰
An acupuncture cavity belonging to the Conception Vessel.

Huo 火
Fire. One of the Five Elements (Wu Xing).

Ji 擠
Press or Squeeze. One of the Four Directions of the eight basic Taiji fighting techniques.

Jin 金
Metal. One of the Five Elements (Wu Xing).

Jin 勁
Power. In Chinese martial arts there are many types of Jin, but they all deal with the flow of energy. These range from sensing Jins (sensing the enemy's power), to neutralizing Jins (neutralizing or deflecting the enemy's power), to emitting Jins (emitting power in a smooth pulse). In general, the higher the level of Jin, the more Qi and the less Li (muscular strength) is used.

Jin Bu 進步
Step Forward. One of the five basic strategic movements of Taiji.

Jing 精
Essence. What is left after something has been refined and purified. In Chinese medicine, Jing can mean semen, but it generally refers to the basic substance of the body which the Qi and Spirit enliven.

Kan 坎
One of the eight trigrams (Bagua). Corresponds to Water.

Kao 靠
Bump. A technique using the shoulder, hip, thigh, back, or any other part of the body to bump the opponent off balance. One of the Four Corners of the eight basic Taiji fighting techniques.

Kao Tao 高濤
Dr. Yang, Jwing-Ming's first Taijiquan master.

Kua 胯
The inner thighs.

Kun 坤
One of the eight trigrams (Bagua). Corresponds to Earth.

Li 力
Muscular power; Strength.

Li 離
One of the eight trigrams (Bagua). Corresponds to Fire.

Li, Mao-Ching 李茂清
Dr. Yang, Jwing-Ming's Long Fist master.

Lie 挒
Split or Rend. The use of two opposing forces to lock or unbalance the opponent. One of the Four Corners of the eight basic Taiji fighting techniques.

Ling 靈
Agile.

Lu 擺
Rollback. A technique for leading the opponent's attack past you. One of the Four Directions of the eight basic Taiji fighting techniques.

Mingmen 命門
Means life door. An acupuncture cavity located on the lower back (between L2 and L3).

Mu 木
Wood. One of the five basic elements (Wu Xing).

Peng 掤
Ward-off. A technique for bouncing the opponent's force back in the direction it came from. One of the Four Directions of the eight basic Taiji fighting techniques.

Qi (Chi) 氣
The "intrinsic energy" which circulates in all living things.

Qi Li (or Li Qi) 氣力 (力氣)
Qi-Supported Muscular Power. When you concentrate your mind (Yi) and keep the muscles relaxed, the Qi flow will increase and invigorate the muscles.

Qian 乾
One of the Eight Trigrams (Bagua). Corresponds to Heaven.

Qigong (Chi Kung) 氣功
A type of Gongfu training which specializes in building up the Qi circulation in the body for health and/or martial purposes.

Qin Na (Chin Na) 擒拿
Grasp and Control. An aspect of Chinese martial arts training, Qin Na specializes in controlling the enemy through "misplacing the bone," "dividing the muscle," "sealing the breath," and "cavity press."

Qing 輕
Lightness.

Qing Ling 輕靈
Lightness and Agility. These words are often used to describe the motion of monkeys—responsive, controlled, and able to move quickly.

Shen 神
Spirit. The consciousness within which the mind and thought function.

Shi 勢
Though commonly translated as "postures," this has the meaning of "the appearance,""the way,""the situation," or "the pattern."

Shuang 雙
Double or Pair.

Shuang Chong 雙重
Double overlapping. This means "mutual covering and resistance" and has the sense of two forces struggling against each other.

Shuang Zhong 雙重
Double Weighting. The fault of not distinguishing between substantial and insubstantial.

Shui 水
Water. One of the five basic elements (Wu Xing).

Sui Xi 髓息
Means "marrow breathing." Through coordination of the breath and the mind, learning to use the mind to lead the Qi to the bone marrow.

Tai Xi 胎息
Embryo breathing. A Qigong breathing technique which can be used to store the Qi in the Real Dan Tian.

Taiji 太極
Grand Ultimate. The state in which opposites (known as Yin and Yang) are generated.

Taiji Jin 太極勁
The martial power manifested in Taijiquan. Usually it means soft Jin.

Taijiquan 太極拳
Grand Ultimate Fist.

Ti Xi 體息
Body breathing. Also called "Fu Xi," which means skin breathing. This is a Qigong breathing technique which allows you to use your mind to lead the Qi to the skin surface, to strengthen the guardian Qi.

Tu 土
Earth. One of the five basic elements (Wu Xing).

Tui Bu 退步
Step Backward. One of the five basic strategic movements of Taijiquan.

Wang, Zong-Yue 王宗岳
A well know Taiji master during the Chinese Qing dynasty.

Wu Bu 五步
Five steppings. The five strategic steppings in Taijiquan thirteen postures.

Wuji 無極

No Extremity. This is the state of undifferentiated emptiness before a beginning. As soon as there is a beginning or a movement, there is differentiation and opposites, and this is called Taiji.

Wushu 武術

Martial Technique. In the beginning, Chinese martial arts were called Wu Yi (Martial Arts), and the techniques of Wu Yi were called Wushu (martial techniques). In 1926, the name was changed to Guoshu (Kuoshu) but was changed back to Wushu in 1949 in China. It is still called Guoshu (Kuoshu) in Taiwan.

Xiao Zhou Tian 小周天

Small Circulation. Nei Dan Qigong training in which Qi is generated at the Dan Tian, and then moved in a circle through the Conception and Governing Vessels.

Xin 心

Heart. In Chinese it often means "mind." It refers to an intention, idea or thought which has not been expressed.

Xun 巽

One of the eight trigrams (Bagua). Corresponds to Wind.

Yang 陽

The positive pole of Taiji (Grand Ultimate), the other pole being Yin (Negative). The Chinese believe that everything follows from the interaction of Yin and Yang.

Yang, Yu-Ting (1887-1982 A.D.) 楊禹廷

A well known Wu style Taijiquan master during the 1960's.

Yang, Jwing-Ming 楊俊敏

Author of this book.

Yi 意

Mind. It is commonly expressed as Xin-Yi. Xin is an idea and Yi is the expression of this idea. Therefore, Yi by itself can be translated as "Mind."

Yi Shou Dan Tian 意守丹田

Means to keep the wisdom mind at the Dan Tian in order to store the Qi.

Yi Yi Yin Qi 以意引氣
Means to use the Yi (wisdom mind) to lead the Qi.

Yin 陰
The negative pole of Taiji (Grand Ultimate). See also Yang.

Yongquan 湧泉
An acupuncture cavity belonging to the Kidney Channel.

You Pan 右盼
Look to the Right. One of the five basic Taiji strategic movements.

Zhang, San-Feng (Chang, San-Feng) 張三豐
Said to be the creator of Taijiquan in the Song Dynasty (960-1279 A.D.). However, there is no certain documentary proof of this.

Zhen 震
One of the eight trigrams (Bagua). Corresponds to Thunder.

Zhong 重
Weight or Heaviness. The same Chinese character, when pronounced as "Chong," means "layering."

Zhong Ding 中定
Central Equilibrium. One of the five basic strategic movements.

Zhou 肘
Elbow. The technique of striking or neutralizing with the elbow. One of the Four Corners of the eight basic Taiji fighting techniques.

Zuo Gu 左顧
Beware of the Left. One of the five fundamental strategic movements which correspond to the Five Elements.

About the Author
Yang, Jwing-Ming, Ph.D.

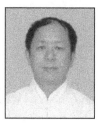

Dr. Yang, Jwing-Ming was born on August 11th, 1946, in *Xinzhu Xian, Taiwan,* Republic of China. He started his *Wushu* (*Gongfu* or *Kung Fu*) training at the age of fifteen under the *Shaolin* White Crane (*Bai He*) Master Cheng, Gin-Gsao. Master Cheng originally learned *Taizuquan* from his grandfather when he was a child. When Master Cheng was fifteen years old, he started learning White Crane from Master Jin, Shao-Feng, and followed him for twenty-three years until Master Jin's death.

In thirteen years of study (1961-1974 A.D.) under Master Cheng, Dr. Yang became an expert in the White Crane Style of Chinese martial arts, which includes both the use of barehands and of various weapons such as saber, staff, spear, trident, two short rods, and many other weapons. With the same master he also studied White Crane *Qigong*, *Qin Na* (or *Chin Na*), *Tui Na* and *Dian Xue* massages, and herbal treatment.

At the age of sixteen, Dr. Yang began the study of *Yang Style Taijiquan* under Master Kao Tao. After learning from Master Kao, Dr. Yang continued his study and research of *Taijiquan* with several masters and senior practitioners such as Master Li, Mao-Ching and Mr. Wilson Chen in *Taipei*. Master Li learned his *Taijiquan* from the well-known Master Han, Ching-Tang, and Mr. Chen learned his *Taijiquan* from Master Zhang, Xiang-San. Dr. Yang has mastered the *Taiji* barehand sequence, pushing hands, the two-man fighting sequence, *Taiji* sword, *Taiji* saber, and *Taiji Qigong*.

When Dr. Yang was eighteen years old he entered Tamkang College in *Taipei Xian* to study Physics. In college he began the study of traditional *Shaolin* Long Fist (*Changquan* or *Chang Chuan*) with Master Li, Mao-Ching at the Tamkang College Guoshu Club (1964-1968 A.D.), and eventually became an assistant instructor under Master Li. In 1971 he completed his M.S. degree in Physics at the National Taiwan University, and then served in the Chinese Air Force from 1971 to 1972. In the service, Dr. Yang taught Physics at the Junior Academy of the Chinese Air Force while also teaching *Wushu*. After being honorably discharged in 1972, he returned to Tamkang College to teach Physics and resumed study under Master Li, Mao-Ching.

From Master Li, Dr. Yang learned Northern Style *Wushu*, which includes both barehand (especially kicking) techniques and numerous weapons.

In 1974, Dr. Yang came to the United States to study Mechanical Engineering at Purdue University. At the request of a few students, Dr. Yang began to teach *Gongfu* (*Kung Fu*), which resulted in the foundation of the Purdue University Chinese Kung Fu Research Club in the spring of 1975. While at Purdue, Dr. Yang also taught college-credited courses in *Taijiquan*. In May of 1978 he was awarded a Ph.D. in Mechanical Engineering from Purdue.

In 1980, Dr. Yang moved to Houston to work for Texas Instruments. While in Houston he founded Yang's Shaolin Kung Fu Academy, which was eventually taken over by his disciple Mr. Jeffery Bolt after Dr. Yang moved to Boston in 1982. Dr. Yang founded Yang's Martial Arts Academy (YMAA) in Boston on October 1, 1982.

In January of 1984 he gave up his engineering career to devote more time to research, writing, and teaching. In March of 1986 he purchased property in the Jamaica Plain area of Boston to be used as the headquarters of the new organization, Yang's Martial Arts Association. The organization has continued to expand, and, as of July 1st 1989,

YMAA has become just one division of Yang's Oriental Arts Association, Inc. (YOAA, Inc.).

In summary, Dr. Yang has been involved in Chinese *Wushu* since 1961. During this time, he has spent thirteen years learning *Shaolin* White Crane (*Bai He*), *Shaolin* Long Fist (*Changquan*), and *Taijiquan*. Dr. Yang has more than twenty-eight years of instructional experience: seven years in Taiwan, five years at Purdue University, two years in Houston, Texas, and fourteen years in Boston, Massachusetts.

In addition, Dr. Yang has also been invited to offer seminars around the world to share his knowledge of Chinese martial arts and *Qigong*. The countries he has visited include Canada, Mexico, France, Italy, Poland, England, Ireland, Portugal, Belgium, Switzerland, Germany, Hungary, Spain, Holland, Latvia, South Africa, and Saudi Arabia.

Since 1986, YMAA has become an international organization, which currently includes over 40 schools located in Poland, Portugal, France, Belgium, Italy, Holland, Hungary, Switzerland, Ireland, United Kingdom, Canada, South Africa, South America and the United States. Many of Dr. Yang's books and videotapes have been translated into languages such as French, Italian, Spanish, Polish, Czech, Bulgarian, Russian, and Hungarian.

Printed in the USA
CPSIA information can be obtained
at www.ICGtesting.com
JSHW021957150824
68134JS00055B/2166